Caesarean Birth

Experience, Practice and History

Helen Churchill, Ph.D.

Senior Lecturer and Health Studies Subject Leader
Crewe+Alsager Faculty
the Manchester Metropolitan University

Books for Midwives Press
An imprint of Hochland & Hochland Ltd

For my caesarean child Leah

Published by Books for Midwives Press, 174a Ashley Road, Hale, Cheshire, WA15 9SF, England

© Helen Churchill, 1997

First edition

ISBN 1-898507-51-1

British Library Cataloguing in Publication Data
A catalogue record for this book is available from the British Library

Printed in Great Britain by Cromwell Press Ltd.

Contents

Acknowledgements

I owe many thanks to many people who have given help, advice and support over the many years that I have been working on this project. To all those people I am very grateful. In particular, I am indebted to Professor Colin Francome of Middlesex University without whose enthusiasm and inspiration this work would not have begun. I am grateful also to Professor Gaye Heathcote, Head of Department, for not only her continued faith in my abilities but also the practical support which she has extended to me.

Thanks and gratitude are extended to the hundreds of women who took part in the studies, giving their time and taking the trouble to fill in the questionnaires while they were still in hospital and probably not feeling at their best. Thanks also to the women who were interviewed and kindly shared their stories, emotions and reactions which enhanced the study. I am very grateful to the consultants, midwives and care managers who organized the distribution and collection of questionnaires in 1991/2 and then agreed to do it all again in 1996. In particular I would like to thank Mr Ian Allen, Mr D. A. Evans, Mrs Pauline Hallam, Mr Roy Husemeyer, Mrs Theresa Lewis, Miss Joan Milne, Mr I. M. Stokes, Miss V. A. Wilkerson and Mrs R Wrigley without whose help and the goodwill of their staff the research would not have been possible.

I extend my warmest gratitude to my family for their continued support, emotionally and practically. Finally, I thank my colleagues at MMU for stepping in at crucial times as research assistants, advisors and counsellors. Finally, a big 'thank you' to Henry Hochland and Catherine Bryant of Hochland & Hochland for their encouragement and enthusiasm for this project.

Some work on the history of caesarean section and aspects of the results of the 1991/92 study into women's experiences of caesarean section have been reprinted with the kind permission of Middlesex University Press. Parts of Chapter Eight were previously published as two articles in the *Nursing Times*.

Introduction

The history of caesarean section is the history of men's achievements (and lack of achievement) with women's bodies. I have researched the origins of the caesarean operation for two reasons. First, because there has been no systematic collection of historical data on the operation since Young published his work over 50 years ago. The study presented here is now the most comprehensive compilation of the history of caesarean section to date. Secondly, to illustrate the attitudes of the medical profession and the development of the medical ethos about women as patients/subjects, to provide the background to the next phase of the work on women's experiences of caesarean birth. It provides a detailed account of the history of the caesarean operation, charting its development from the earliest times and examining the diverse indications that have been identified as necessitating the performance of the operation. The early chapters highlight the fact that interventions in childbirth, particularly the caesarean section, have always been contentious, it is the reasoning behind the debates that have changed over time.

High rates of caesarean section in the late twentieth century have not led to improvements in maternal or infant outcome, and may be responsible for iatrogenic morbidity and mortality. The increased use of abdominal delivery together with other interventionist techniques have had a deleterious effect on women's experience of delivery and denied them the opportunity to achieve a sense of accomplishment in childbirth. The aim of this study was to elicit responses from women having caesareans on a range of issues associated with their experiences of operative birth, in order to provide a detailed analysis of women's experience of caesarean section, and, ultimately, to suggest ways in which the outcome of surgical birth can be improved for women, their babies and hospital staff.

Chapter One examines some theories on the origin of the term 'caesarean section' and looks at references to the operation in myth and folklore. The early history of abdominal delivery is covered here, dating back to 3000 BC. An account of caesarean section during the sixteenth and seventeenth centuries introduces the debate amongst the medical fraternity over the relative benefits and disadvantages of performing the operation. During pre-industrial times the Church had an influence on the decision-making of most aspects of life including pregnancy and childbirth. Thus, the role of the Church in relation to the caesarean operation is introduced in this chapter.

Chapter Two covers the history of caesarean section during the eighteenth century. Despite some improvements in success rates (success being judged in terms of maternal survival), the important debate over the propriety of performing the operation continued, one school of thought believing that it was a necessary course of action when a woman could not deliver vaginally, the other viewing the caesarean as tantamount to murder. This is not surprising considering the very high, practically total, maternal mortality rate that accompanied the operation during its early history.

Chapter Three covers caesareans in the nineteenth century and demonstrates that by the end of the eighteenth century there had been a polarization of attitudes towards the caesarean between French and British obstetricians. The French viewing the operation as preferable to leaving women with difficult labours to the rigours of nature, or resorting to the destruction of the infant, whilst the British view remained sternly opposed to caesareans. This chapter also gives details of maternal and infant mortality figures associated with the operation at that time.

Chapter Four reviews the procedures, other than the caesarean section, that were developed to aid delivery during the eighteenth and nineteenth centuries. Some techniques, such as the symphyseotomy, were designed to supersede the caesarean. Others, for example, induction of premature labour, were proposed in order to pre-empt the necessity for abdominal delivery. Craniotomy was the method preferred by the British obstetricians who opposed the use of caesarean section.

Chapter Five examines the evidence available on self-inflicted caesareans, that is, women performing the operation on themselves. The earliest recorded case occurred during the eighteenth century, although the phenomena is not entirely unheard of in the twentieth century. In the majority of cases the outcome of the operation was not good for the infant. However, evidence suggests that throughout much of its history the practice of self-inflicted caesarean was actually safer for women than the so-called 'professional' procedures.

Chapter Six charts the development of the operative technique for the caesarean section. From the early stages in development when each operation could have been as individual as the surgeon performing it, to more recent times when the precise technique for performing the operation has been clearly documented, revised and updated. Included in this chapter are details of important contributions to improvements in technique introduced by Porro and Sanger, together with the historical background to the, now familiar, lower-segment operation. The chapter ends with a brief summary of changes in the main indications for caesarean section up until the twentieth century.

Chapter Seven details the role played by the caesarean operation in childbirth practice in the twentieth century. The concept of 'once a caesarean, always a caesarean', which continues to affect section rates today, is introduced here. The chapter demonstrates that decreases in maternal mortality associated with the procedure led to increases in caesarean section rates, to the extent that the number of operations performed became a cause for concern. An issue which continues to be contentious.

Chapter Eight sets the scene for the study of the modern caesarean by examining the concept of 'conflict' in maternity care by exposing the differing perceptions and experiences of childbirth between women and obstetricians. Notions of 'success', 'satisfaction' and 'knowledge' are examined in relation to childbirth, together with an important debate on the issue of 'power'. Knowledge and information are crucial determinants in the distribution of power between women and doctors and their role in this important relationship are assessed in this chapter.

Chapter Nine provides a background for the empirical stage of the study by highlighting current trends in caesarean section rates and examining the influences which affect differences in those rates. An international comparison is given together with a discussion of the influence of caesarean rates on perinatal and neonatal outcomes.

Chapter Ten begins with a descriptive account of medical indications for the caesarean operation today. It then examines non-medical variables, such as fear of litigation and consultant preference, which affect the number of operations performed. The evidence presented in this chapter suggests that too many caesareans are carried out for non-medical reasons and that this has serious implications for women in childbirth.

Chapter Eleven examines the effects of caesarean section on women, their babies and the mother-child relationship. Relative benefits of the type of anaesthesia and operation (emergency or elective) are discussed here, together with evidence suggesting that elective operations performed under regional anaesthetic reduce negative sequelae in caesarean patients.

Chapter Twelve gives details of empirical work undertaken for the current study into women's experiences of caesarean birth. The section begins with a statement of the theory of the research together with the hypotheses and research questions. An account of the methodology is given followed by precise details of the results of two studies, 1991/2 and 1996.

Chapter Thirteen provides a discussion of the results in relation to the first hypothesis, examining whether women suffer as a result of caesarean section. The results demonstrate that women do suffer following abdominal delivery, both psychologically and physically, and that these effects can have a damaging consequences for the mother-child relationship.

Chapter Fourteen concludes the thesis by examining the second hypothesis which concerns improvements in maternity services. The chapter summarizes the main findings of the study and details recommendations on how the practice of caesarean section can be improved to ensure a better outcome for women and their babies as well as hospital staff.

CHAPTER ONE

Caesareans in Pre-Industrial Times

Caesarean section: myth and folklore

There have been many myths about caesareans in literature and folklore and the origin of the term 'caesarean section' has been the subject of much debate. One suggestion is that the term caesarean was derived from the birth of Julius Caesar or one of his ancestors who is said to have been delivered in this way. Yet the birth of Julius Caesar is unlikely to have been by this method as there are no recorded maternal survivals following caesarean birth at that time (100–144 BC) and Julius Caesar's mother lived on long after his birth (Newell, 1921). This, coupled with the fact that the term 'caesarean birth' was not recorded to have been used until 1581, suggests that the association of the caesarean operation with Julius Caesar is likely to be a myth.

It is reputed that a law was passed in Rome in 715 BC by the King, Numa Pompilius, forbidding the burial of a pregnant woman upon her death until the fetus had been removed in order that the mother and child could be buried separately. The caesarean operation was thus mandatory in such cases. Newell, writing in 1921, suggested that this offered an explanation for the origin of the term 'caesarean'. The Roman law, the 'Lex Regia' became the 'Lex Cesaria' and thus the practice became known as the caesarean operation.

An alternative explanation was proposed by Delee (1913) who suggested that the word 'caesarean' comes from the Latin 'caesaru' meaning 'to cut'. The word was first used in connection with this operation by a French physician, Rousset in 1581 (Young, 1944). The word 'section' (Latin: 'seco') also implies cutting and can mean 'incision'. But 'incision' can be interpreted as 'to part' or 'to divide' which refers to the process of 'opening'. If Delee's theory is correct, the term 'caesarean section' literally means either 'cut cut' (meaning that the combined use of these words as in the British use of the term 'caesarean section' is unnecessary) or, a more plausible translation of the term caesarean section is 'cut open'.

Robert II, King of Scotland, is reputed to have been born by caesarean section on the 2nd of March, 1316. The operation was carried out postmortem following the death of his mother from a broken neck after falling from her horse. There is also speculation that Edward VI, son of Henry VIII and Jane Seymour, may have been delivered by caesarean on October 12th, 1537. There is some confusion as to the exact number of days the Queen survived after the birth and also whether she was already dying during labour or died because of the operation. The King is reputed to have ordered the caesarean section to be carried out when asked by the attending physicians whether to save the life of the infant at the risk losing his wife. The King's reason being that he could always replace his wife! (Hull, 1798).[1]

Various myths and legends from different regions suggest that abdominal birth was widely believed to be the 'godly' way to enter the world. A person who had been cut out of her/his mother's body was considered to be 'unborn' until the eighteenth century (Lomas and Enkin, 1989).

Shakespeare mentioned the caesarean operation in his play Macbeth. In a desperate attempt to save his own life, Macbeth declares that he 'must not yield to one of woman born'. Unfortunately, this tactic is rendered useless when his assailant, Macduff, declares that he was born by caesarean, or rather, 'from his mothers womb, Untimely ripped' (Shakespeare, 1605).

Caesarean section in pre-industrial times

It is impossible to ascertain when the caesarean section was first performed. The antiquity of the operation, however, is definitely established under the early Roman civilizations. Records show that as early as 3000 BC in Egypt and 1500 BC in India among the ancient Hindus, the removal of the fetus by a surgical incision of the abdomen was mandatory by law at the time of death of the mother if movement of the fetus was detectable (known as post-mortem caesarean). It appears that the operation was rarely, if ever, carried out on a living woman. The earliest record of a child surviving the operation is that of a Sicilian orator, Gorgias, in 508 BC (Young, 1944).

The caesarean section is recorded to have been performed on the wife of a Tartar prince in China during the Wei dynasty (AD 225). Both mother and child are reputed to have survived (Bishop, 1960).

It is probable that the operation was known to the early Jews as it was mentioned in the 'Mischnagoth' (the oldest book of Judaism) which was first published in 140 BC and possibly earlier. The operation also appeared in the 'Talmud' (the next oldest book which originated between the second and sixth centuries). In fact among this religious group it must have been carried out on living women who were expected to survive as their law stated that women having caesareans were not required to observe days of purification as did those who had a vaginal delivery (Bishop, 1960). However there is some scepticism regarding the use of caesarean section by the early Jews:

> 'Several authorities believe that certain passages in the Talmud may be so interpreted as to point to its performance on the living amongst the Jews, but the evidence is, to say the least, unconvincing and lacking in authority.' (Newell, 1921, p. 3)

---

1. Despite having been acknowledged by a number of writers, it was recorded in the eighteenth century that both of these events lack evidence and are therefore without foundation (Hull, 1798).

The extent to which the operation was performed is unknown but, despite the doubts of commentators such as Newell, the limited evidence available does suggest that it is extremely likely that the caesarean section was practiced long before the start of the Christian era.

One of the most famous figures of the medical history of India during the fifth century was Susruta. His extensive lists of the methods and instruments of surgery included the caesarean section (Bishop, 1960), thus confirming that the operation was known to early civilizations in India.

The early Christian era is likely to have had an effect on the practice of the caesarean section. It appears that from early Christian times to the sixteenth century, the caesarean section was hardly used at all. When it was employed, it was more often practiced in cases where the woman had died late in pregnancy in the hope of saving the child (Newell, 1921).

Caesareans in the sixteenth and seventeenth centuries

In more recent history it is recorded that in 1542 a surgeon, Maitre Vincent, performed the operation on a woman, Nicole Beranger. The child was already dead but the patient made a full recovery and later gave birth to two children vaginally (Young, 1944). If this information is correct, it is of utmost importance because it represents the first delivery by caesarean section with a recorded maternal survival.

The next maternal survival from a caesarean was not recorded until almost 50 years later. It is reputed that Jacob Nufer, a Swiss hog gelder, performed a caesarean section on his wife, Elizabeth Alespachin, during a prolonged and obstructed labour in Sigerhausen, Switzerland in 1588. Mother and child survived and recovered. Elizabeth went on to deliver six more children, one set of twins and four single births, presumably vaginally, and the child, despite her/his dramatic entrance to the world, is reputed to have lived to the age of 77 (related in Caspar Bauhin's Appendix to 'Rousset's Treatise', 1588, from Hull, 1798; The Lancet, 1851a; Newell, 1921). This event is highly significant in the history of the caesarean section as it is the first recorded case of the operation where both mother and child survived.

The debate: To section or not to section?

It was during the sixteenth century that the debate over the ethicacy of performing the operation on a living woman began. One school of thought believing that the mother's life could be saved in the event of obstructed labour by surgical removal of the child, and the other seeing the operation as tantamount to murder. A determined opponent of the operation was Ambrose Paré (1510–1590) who condemned those who would dare to perform it because 'no man can persuade me [it] can be done without the death of the mother' (Paré, 1579, translated 1678, in Young, 1944, p. 24).

The term 'caesarean birth' was first used by the Frenchman Rousset in 1581. Although he had not performed the operation himself, his paper was important because it opened the debate on the relative benefits of the operation and drew attention to the possibility of performing the caesarean on a living woman (Young, 1944). The debate continued and in a book on midwifery published in 1856, Scipione Mercurio described the caesarean operation suggesting that it was feasible on a living woman. However, he urged caution saying that it should only be used as a last resort and following careful consideration of the woman's physical state (Thoms, 1935). In another book on childbirth, published by Guillimeau in 1598, the usefulness of performing the operation on a living woman was discussed but Guillimeau did not advocate the practice. He had performed the operation twice in the presence of Ambrose Paré and some of the most distinguished surgeons of Paris. Both women died (The Lancet, 1851a). Guillimeau stated that in 1609 he had witnessed the operation performed on three other women and they also had died. In recounting Guillimeau's work, *The Lancet*, some 240 years later, suggested that these disastrous results lead to the abandonment of the caesarean operation by all 'sound' (sic) practitioners in Paris (The Lancet, 1851a).

The work of Scipione Mercurio (1540–1616) was important to the caesarean debate of the late sixteenth century. Not only was he one of the first to publish the exact procedure for the operation but he also advocated the use of sutures to secure the abdominal wound (Thoms, 1935). Furthermore, Mercurio became the first surgeon to advocate the caesarean section for cases of contracted pelvis in 1604 (Young, 1944). This was important because it implied for the first time that the medical or physical condition of the woman prior to labour may have an effect on her experience during labour, a fact which had not been publicly considered before.

On April 21st 1610, Professor Sennert of Wittenberg University recorded a case of a caesarean section being performed by Trautmann on a woman for whom a natural delivery was impossible because of a large hernia containing the pregnant uterus (Newell, 1921). According to Young (1944), this operation represented:

> 'The first definitely authentic case of caesarean section intentionally performed upon a living woman.' (p. 30)

Unfortunately the woman died 25 days after the operation from an infection because the surgeon had not closed the wound or the uterus. Such omission was common at that time.

The high maternal mortality rate associated with caesarean section is not surprising considering that the operation was a very rudimentary procedure during the sixteenth and seventeenth centuries. Anaesthetics had not been developed and so the woman remained awake and fully aware during the operation. The patient would be tied down or held by assistants. The wounds in the uterus and the abdomen were frequently not sutured but left gaping. The external wound may occasionally be brought together by a couple of crude stitches or bandages.

Thus the performing of the operation on a living woman remained highly controversial and in 1616 William Harvey (renowned for discovering the circulation of the blood) followed his predecessors in stating that the caesarean operation should only be used on the death of the mother (Young, 1944).

One of the early champions of the caesarean section was Hendrik van Roonhuyze. In 1663 he published what has been described as the first work in operative gynaecology. In it he cited the case of Sonnius, a physician of Bruges, who had performed the operation several times on his wife, obviously with a great deal of success. Roonhuyze himself was also noted as having successfully performed the operation (Young, 1944).

Considering the high (practically total) maternal mortality rate associated with the caesarean section, success was judged in terms of survival of the mother. Success, however, was a rare event and so the debate over the propriety of performing the operation continued. Francois Mauriceau (1637–1709) published a book in 1668 on pregnancy and childbirth, translated by Chamberlen in 1672, which soon became the textbook of English accoucheurs (The Lancet, 1851a), and was apparently the most thorough and well-informed work produced at that time (Young, 1944). As one of the leading obstetricians of the seventeenth century, Mauriceau's determined opposition to the caesarean section, except in post-mortem cases, became one of the biggest obstacles to the development of the operation at that time. His argument was that as the operation meant almost certain death to the mother, surgeons had no right to determine that a mother should die in order to save the life of her child. He stated:

> 'I do not know if there was ever any law, Christian or Civil, which doth ordain the martyring and killing of the mother to save the child.' (Mauriceau in Lomas and Enkin, 1989, p. 1183)

It is difficult to estimate the number of caesarean sections being performed in pre-industrial times with any degree of certainty. From the sixteenth to the nineteenth century the statistics on the performance of caesareans were fragmentary and in some ways contradictory. Churchill recorded that in the sixteenth century there were 24 successful cases of caesarean section. In the seventeenth century there were 33 operations and only 8 fatalities (Churchill, 1841, in Young, 1944). Young offers an explanation for the low fatality rate as, not competence in the operative technique, but rather, enthusiasm for reporting successful cases and reluctance to report unsuccessful operations (1944). This is not surprising given the violent opposition to the operation from many of the leading obstetricians in Britain at that time.

The role of the Church – part I

During pre-industrial times religion played a leading role in the decision-making of most aspects of life including pregnancy and childbirth. The Roman Catholic Church barred abortions, craniotomy or embryotomy as measures for delivering the fetus in order to save the life of the mother. In 1733 the medical profession asked the doctors of theology at the Sorbonne whether it was religiously correct to sacrifice the woman in order to possibly save the life of the baby in the case where a woman could not deliver vaginally. On March 30th they replied that if one could only save the life of one or the other there was a conflict. Justice would imply it better to sacrifice the baby. However, they believed that according to charity it was better to save the baby because it was only at the expense of the mother's life that the baptism of the child be assured and eternal life therefore secured (Young, 1944). This ruling meant that craniotomy was not allowable in order to save the life of the mother. It was their view that the child must be removed in order that it may be baptized to save it from having to spend eternity in 'limbo', a place in between heaven and hell that once existed in the official doctrines of the Church. Sacrifice of the mother's life was justifiable as she had already been baptized and would therefore avoid such an unspeakable fate (Guillimeau, 1612). The fetus in utero was seen to have two kinds of life – a corporeal (or bodily) one, the other a spiritual life. The latter only being endowed on the fetus through baptism. The spiritual life of the child was regarded as more precious than the corporeal life of the mother (The Lancet, 1851a). Thus the question of whether or not to perform the caesarean operation ceased to be a purely obstetrical, surgical or scientific one and became strictly a theological one.

The Church also advocated caesarean section in the case where the woman had died (Newell, 1921). This is comparable to the earlier practices in ancient civilizations as discussed above but the reasoning was different. The Catholic view was, again, to save the soul of the child. Guillimeau (1612) stressed the importance of the operation 'that thereby the child may be saved and receive baptism' (p. 224), although he was not advocating sacrifice of the mother's life for this purpose. He stated:

> 'Lawyers judge them worthy of death, who shall bury a great bellied woman that is dead before the child is taken forth because they seem to destroy the hope of a living creature. The chirurgion must be certainly assured that the woman is dead, and that her kinsfolk, friends and others that are present, do all affirm that her soul is departed.' (p. 185)

He continued to say that to be assured that the mother had in fact died, one should place some light feathers over her mouth and with even light breath they would fly away.

Thus the caesarean section is not a modern endeavour. The operation was certainly known to, and practiced in early civilizations. However, it appears that throughout most of its early history, the operation was carried out post mortem, as a last resort, either in an attempt to save the life of the child, or because of religious dictate which called for the separation of mother and child. The high maternal mortality rate which accompanied the surgery meant that it was rarely carried out on living women as this would mean almost certain death.

CHAPTER TWO

Caesareans in the Eighteenth Century

From the early eighteenth century, doctors became increasingly involved in childbirth with a resultant surge in publications on obstetrics. The numbers of caesareans being performed slowly increased and successful cases were accounted in great detail. Success again was measured in terms of maternal survival. As detailed previously, some earlier attempts had managed to save the child but had resulted in maternal death in most cases.

In the early part of the century Ruleau published a dissertation discussing the usefulness of the caesarean section and also describing a successful operation he had performed on a patient who had been in labour for five days. Both the mother and child survived (Ruleau, 1704, in Young, 1944). Similarly, the use of the caesarean operation was (somewhat cautiously) advised by Guillaume de la Motte in 1721, particularly for cases of extreme distortion of the pelvis, thus advocating the use of the operation on living women (de la Motte, 1721, in Young, 1944). Supporting this view later that decade, Simon, a French surgeon, furthered the cause of the caesarean operation stating that the procedure should be carried out where vaginal delivery was impossible. He supported this claim with the description of eleven successful cases carried out between 1723 and 1738 (Young, 1944).

However, there were some relentless opponents to the operation. Dionis published a work on obstetrics in 1718 stating that under no circumstances should the operation be performed unless the woman was dead, and that anyone who would operate on a living woman deserves to be punished for their butchery. In Britain too, opposition to the operation continued and in 1739, Sir Richard Manningham advised that as the operation was always fatal (sic) to the mother it should only be performed after her death (Manningham, 1739, in Young, 1944). This being the most popular opinion on caesarean section at that time, midwives were likewise advised to only perform the operation on a patient who had died. The rules of midwifery contained instructions on how to ascertain whether or not the mother had actually expired so that the caesarean could be carried out: 'If she does not respond to penetrating odor (sic), is ice-cold, without pulse, looks collapsed and pale as death, and if her breath leaves no traces on a mirror' (Nöth, 1913, p. 84), then, presumably, the woman could be considered dead and the operation performed.

The first recorded caesarean section to be carried out in Great Britain was performed by Smith, an Edinburgh surgeon on 29th June 1737, when summoned to a patient who had been in labour for six days. On examining the patient he found that a normal delivery was impossible and performed the caesarean section with the agreement of two other physicians and the relatives of the patient who had been duly warned of the risks involved. The child was removed dead and the woman died the following day (Young, 1944). This experience clearly did not silence the critics of the operation.

Seven months later, on the 1st January 1738, the first recorded caesarean section performed by a midwife, Mary Donally, in the then United Kingdom was performed. The patient was Alice O'Neale, aged 33, of Charlemont, Ireland, mother of several children. Alice had been in labour for 12 days and attended by numerous midwives with no success. The child was believed to be dead after the third day. In desperation relatives called in a local woman famous among the community for extracting dead infants, Mary Donally. After attempting to deliver the patient without success she performed a caesarean operation. On removing the dead infant Mary Donally held the sides of the wound together with her hands while neighbours went to fetch silk and a tailor's needle with which she stitched the wound. Donally then treated the wound with the white of eggs. Alice O'Neale made a full recovery but later developed a large ventral hernia as did many other patients of caesarean section at that time (Stewart, 1771).

Duncan Stewart, a surgeon from Dungannon, County Tyrone, Ireland, wrote:

> 'In about twenty seven days the patient was able to walk a mile on foot, and came to me in a farmer's house, where she showed me the wound covered with a cicatrice, but she complained of her belly hanging outwards on the right side where I... advised to support the side of her belly with a bandage. The patient has enjoyed good health ever since, manages her family affairs, and has frequently walked to market in this town which is six miles distance from her own house.' (Stewart, 1747, pp. 361–62)

The fact that the first successful operation in Great Britain was performed by a midwife did not please the medical profession and in the literature there was much disparagement of midwife Donally's success. In 1855 Dr. Robert Lee was reported in *The Lancet* as calling Mary Donally an 'ignorant Irish midwife'. He then went on to cast doubts over whether the case actually existed and suggested that it should be removed from the data on successful cases (The Lancet, 1851a, p. 154). In the most comprehensive account of the history of the caesarean section up to the middle of this century, Young called Mary Donally's achievement 'a matter of good luck rather than good judgement' (Young, 1944, p. 54), thereby demonstrating a continued reluctance to acknowledge the skill of this midwife. More recently an account in a British midwifery journal stated of this event: '...since no qualified person attended the delivery or witnessed the events, it has generally been discounted' (Frazer, 1987, p. 73). However, Stewart, the surgeon who examined the patient in the puerperium clearly believed the account, as did Smellie, one of the most influential obstetricians of the eighteenth century (1766).

In 1742, the *Treatise of Midwifery* by Fielding Ould was published. This work condemned the caesarean operation suggesting that any dilemma about whether the life of the mother is worth risking in an attempt to save the life of the child could only be answered by the 'Divines' (Ould, 1742, in Young, 1944).

The great debate

By the mid-eighteenth century few members of the medical profession were prepared to speak out in favour of the operation. One of the few was John Burton who, in 1751, became the first British obstetrician to write in support of the caesarean section despite not having performed the operation himself. As only an extremely limited number of caesareans had been performed in Britain at that time, Burton presumably based his work on the writings of the French obstetricians. In his book, Burton went into the greatest detail on the caesarean section than had been previously undertaken. Burton believed that the operation was necessary in certain cases and that the risks associated with the process had been exaggerated by previous writers (Burton, 1751, in Young, 1944). His views were not well received, which is not surprising given the strength of opinion against the operation in Britain at that time.

Two years later, in 1753, a work that was more favourably received than Burton's was published by William Smellie. In *A Treatise on the Theory and Practice of Midwifery*, Smellie took the more conservative view of caesarean section with regards to living patients, that is, as a last resort, performed only on a woman who is strong and healthy and cannot possibly be delivered by any other method. Otherwise, according to Smellie, the usefulness of the operation was limited to attempting to save the life of the infant following the death of the mother (Smellie, 1766).

It was also during the latter half of the eighteenth century that the first suggestion was made that the caesarean section could be used by obstetricians for personal rather than medical reasons (an argument which continues today). In 1783, William Dease condemned the operation stating that in many cases it had been performed unnecessarily by rash and ignorant men anxious to establish a reputation. He declared that 'much to the honour of the Irish surgeons' the operation had never been performed in Dublin (Dease, 1783, in Young, 1944, p. 49).

In the same year, Alexander Hamilton, Professor of Midwifery at Edinburgh University, published the first edition of his major work on obstetrics *Outlines of the Theory and Practice of Midwifery* in which he conceded that caesarean section was necessary in cases of contracted pelvis, but only:

> 'when it appears absolutely impossible to deliver the woman by any other means... we ought then only to employ the dreadful expedient of cutting into the uterus to extract the child.' (Hamilton, 1783, in Young, 1944, p. 52)

However, he was later to argue very strongly against the operation and recommend craniotomy as preferable to caesarean section in most cases (Hamilton, 1803).

Thus strong opposition to the operation continued, based mainly on the extremely high maternal mortality rates associated with it. Aitken (1785) stated:

> 'this formidable operation, intended to save mother and child, has been performed during many centuries with various success. In Britain it has never fully had the desired effect, all the mothers have died.' (Aitken, 1785, in Lomas and Enkin, 1989, p. 1183)

Writing in 1788, Jaques Rene Tenon recorded only 79 successful caesarean sections in the whole of Europe since 1500 (Tenon, 1788). This number reflected the great risk involved in the operation at that time. In 1792, Osborn called the caesarean section a most 'fatal operation'. Being equally opposed to the symphyseotomy, Osborn recommended performing craniotomy early in labour (Osborn, 1792, in Young 1944, p. 51).

The success rate rises

It was not until 1793 that James Barlow, a surgeon of Blackburn, Lancashire, carried out the first successful caesarean section recorded in this country to have been performed by a physician. His patient, Jane Foster, had an extremely deformed pelvis due to being run over by a loaded cart prior to becoming pregnant. When she went into labour she understandably became very distressed and was in much pain. As normal delivery was impossible, caesarean section was suggested and the likely outcome of the operation explained to the patient. Her pain and distress being considerable by this time, Jane Foster agreed with little hesitation. The operation was performed with no anaesthetic, the wound was stitched and then the patient wrapped in flannel. Both mother and child are reputed to have survived (Barlow, 1822).

The following year (1794), the first successful caesarean section in the United States was recorded to have been carried out in a log cabin in Edom, Kanawha Valley, Virginia. Doctor Jesse Bennett performed the operation on his wife in a frontier settlement. Labour was difficult due to a contracted pelvis and Doctor Alex Humphrey was called in for consultation. Forceps failed and Mrs Bennett did not want a craniotomy. Doctor Humphrey would not perform the caesarean and so Doctor Bennett did it himself. Mrs Bennett was stretched out on a crude plank resting on two barrels and put under the influence of a large dose of opium. Both mother and child survived. Doctor Bennett refused to report the procedure in the medical literature as he felt that no one would believe that both mother and child survived (Cianfrani, 1960, in NIH, 1981). However it appears that his fears were unfounded as the *Journal of the American Medical Association* (JAMA) at the time stated dramatically:

> 'The courageous frontier surgeon by one quick stroke of the knife opened the abdomen and uterus and quickly delivered the child and placenta. At this stage he delayed long enough to remove the ovaries. The wounds were closed by a stout linen thread and contrary to the expectations of everyone present Mrs Bennett was soon well and active.' (JAMA, 1794, p. 1942)

Back in London at that time, the debate among the obstetricians raged on. Thomas Denman published his *Introduction to the Practise of Midwifery*. He agreed with Hamilton that caesarean section should only be performed in cases of severe deformity of the pelvis and that the decision to operate should not be made by one practitioner but in consultation with as many practitioners as possible (Denman, 1794, in Young, 1944, p. 53). It was Thomas Denman who continued the discussion on the ethical issue of saving the child at the expense of the mother's life, a course which he believed could be justified. His rationale for such action being that if repeated attempts to deliver a live child had been frustrated by a restricted pelvis, the parents could possibly be offered the option of caesarean section as a means of fulfilling 'one great end of marriage', that is, procreation, even if this meant the probable death of the mother! (Denman, 1794, in Young, 1944, p. 50).

The caesarean controversy

In 1798, Dr John Hull became the first person recorded to have carried out more than one caesarean. As with his first attempt, only the child survived. Further, 1798 marked the beginning of an important controversy over the caesarean section operation between Dr Hull and Mr W. Simmons, both of Manchester. Simmons published a paper entitled 'Reflections on the Propriety of Performing the Caesarean Operation' (1798) in which he highlighted the very high (practically total) fatality rate from the operation in England compared to the relatively good success rates recorded for the rest of Europe. Not believing the rates for other countries to be of relevance to England he advocated the traditional conservative use of the operation only in the event of the death of the mother. Hull took exception to Simmons' condemnation of caesarean section and in a reply paper later that month he pointed out many discrepancies in Simmons' argument against the operation, not least of all his assertion that it was always fatal to the mother (Hull, 1798).

Hull published a book in that year entitled *A Defence of the Cesarean Operation* in which he questioned whether the operation was always fatal to the mother and went on to list the situations in which he would recommend the use of the operation:

'1.   where the Mother is dead, for the preservation of her Offspring;
2.   where the Child is dead, or supposed to be so, for the preservation of the Parent;
3.   where the Mother and Child are living, for the preservation of both.'
(Hull, 1798, p. 5)

In his book, Hull quoted Simmons as saying that the caesarean:

'has proved fatal in England in every instance... [and is] an operation that has proved so fatal to my country women... [that it] must be abandoned.' (Simmons, 1798, in Hull, 1798, p. 7)

Hull went to great lengths to point out the difference between the patient '*dying from an operation*, and *after an operation*' (Hull, 1798, p. 8, original emphasis). Hull accused Simmons of being 'blinded by prejudice' and suggested that he had made his judgement on cases without knowledge of the full facts and conditions of the patient in each case and as such 'the value of the operation ought to be appreciated' for such cases (Hull, 1798, pp. 8–10).

Following a response from Simmons in May 1799, Hull once again defended the caesarean section operation and went on to write one of the most comprehensive lists of circumstances which may necessitate the use of the operation. Most of his 'indications' revolved around variations of restricted pelvis and also included uterine rapture, abnormal presentation, deformity of the fetus and extra-uterine gestation (Hull, 1799, in Young, 1944). Hull's writings have been referred to as the most valuable and illuminating to the medical profession at the time (Young, 1944).

Simmons responded to Hull's work following the death of a woman, Elizabeth Thompson, in Manchester after a caesarean operation performed by Mr Wood. The theme of Simmons' response was that to perform the operation on a living woman was tantamount to murder. Throughout his writings Simmons upheld the notion that only God is able to decide who should live and who should die and that it was not up to physicians to make this choice (Simmons, 1799, in Young, 1944).

The debate which took place between Hull and Simmons is an important one in the history of caesarean section because it highlighted the relative advantages and disadvantages of performing the operation. As Radford (1865) stated, the controversy 'brought the greater part of the medical profession to entertain more clear and definite opinions' (p. 1). However, the balance of opinion in Britain, contrary to that in France, remained against the operation.

Up to the end of the eighteenth century, Radford recorded that there had been nineteen caesarean section operations performed by physicians in Britain. Of the nineteen operations, only two mothers and seven children had survived. However, he was of the opinion that this figure was remarkable considering that the operation was such a 'hazardous undertaking' at that time. Before the 1800s caesarean sections had been 'operations of desperation' performed as a last resort on dying mothers, in an attempt to save the baby. Those surgeons who dared to perform the operation were most often treated with scorn and condemnation by their British colleagues (Radford, 1865, p. 11). Thus by the end of the eighteenth century the caesarean remained a controversial issue and few obstetricians would actually attempt the operation.

CHAPTER THREE

Caesareans in the Nineteenth Century

During the nineteenth century the debate over whether 'to section or not to section' raged on.

The year 1798 was very important in deciding the future of policy for performing caesareans throughout the nineteenth century. It ended with doctors in Britain and France making different decisions about the operation.

French optimism

French proponents of the caesarean section, such as Baudelocque, were eager to point out that despite the hazards, the fate awaiting the patient if the operation was not performed could have been much more horrific (Baudelocque, 1801). In a report to the Society of Medicine in Paris (September 1798) he stated:

> 'In order to admit the necessity of this operation, it ought to be demonstrated, that there is more advantage in performing it, or less risk incurred by the woman, than in leaving her and her child to the efforts of nature, as has been usually done to this very time.' (1801, p. 19)

Baudelocque made an influential contribution to the caesarean section debate in his *Memoirs on Caesarean Section* (1798 and 1799, translated by Hull in 1801). The aim of his first paper was to raise a number of questions:

> '1st.   Do cases exist, in which delivery by the natural passages is physically impossible?
> 2nd.   These cases being determined to exist, is the caesarean operation indispensably necessary?
> 3rd.   Is the caesarean operation inevitably fatal to the mother?' (p. 9)

Baudelocque accepted the necessity of the operation for cases of contracted pelvis and other unusual conditions, and went on to add the condition of tumours of the vagina as an indication. He therefore highlighted the fact that there are some cases where vaginal delivery is absolutely impossible and caesarean section the only option available to extract the child. Baudelocque was critical of other interventionist techniques such as craniotomy, symphyseotomy and induction, suggesting that laws needed to be passed obliging obstetricians to carry out caesarean section in certain circumstances rather than outlawing its practice as some of his predecessors had proposed (Baudelocque, 1801).

After a discussion of Baudelocque's report, the Society of Medicine in Paris accepted that the operation had been a success and in some cases could lead to saving the lives of both the mother and baby. It unanimously decided that it was the duty of the physician to carry out caesareans and that two hundred extra copies of Baudelocque's report should be sent to different judicial and administrative bodies (Baudelocque, 1801). There was some opposition outside the Society, notably from a colourful character called Jean Francis Saccombe who had studied in England under William Hunter, the best known of the contemporary British obstetricians. Saccombe, who founded the 'Ecole Anti-Caesarienne' (anti-caesarean school) in 1798, made the bold claim that he could deliver any woman without resorting to the use of instruments, by virtue of his hands alone. An avid anti-caesareanist, Saccombe denounced pro-caesareanists such as Baudelocque as murderers. Believing the healing of a uterine incision to be unlikely, he claimed that those who practiced caesarean section did so for their own personal gain in terms of finance and publicity (Young, 1944). Not surprisingly, Saccombe was fined 3,000 Francs for slander of Baudelocque and later fled the country.

British conservatism

In Britain the anti-caesarean lobby was in ascendance and led to a difference in practice from the rest of Europe. At the beginning of the nineteenth century, the bulk of British obstetric opinion was opposed to caesareans and the textbooks of the time reflected that view. In 1803, Alexander Hamilton published the fifth edition of his book entitled *Outlines of the Theory and Practice of Midwifery* in which he argued against the major indications commonly used to identify the necessity for the operation at that time. His reasoning was thus:

1. Blocked or contracted passages
Hamilton stated that in cases where the usual delivery passage was blocked by tumours, for instance, it was never necessary to perform the caesarean section. He stressed that tumours of the vagina could be removed in safety even after labour had commenced, and further suggested the possibility of passing a hand by the side of the tumour to turn the child and deliver. He believed that as long as no deformity of the pelvis was present, the child could be delivered in the usual way through the force of the contractions or the use of the scalpel to remove obstacles.

2. Lacerated uterus
According to Hamilton, these cases were usually fatal and could not be saved by caesarean section. He argued against the operation, saying that it was inhumane to perform it on a dying mother even if the rationale was to save the life of the child. Rather, he suggested, one should wait at least until the mother 'expires' (p. 263).

3. Ventral conception (conception outside of the womb/uterus, for example, ectopic)
Hamilton suggested that despite the pain to the mother, the expulsion of such pregnancies should be 'generally trusted to nature' (p. 266).

4. Uterine hernias
Hamilton stated that hernias were not sufficient indication to necessitate the performance of the caesarean section and that deliveries under such circumstances have been happily performed 'without recourse having been made to so hazardous an expedient' (p. 266).

5. Position or size of the child
Hamilton dismissed caesarean section for such cases believing the operation to be totally unnecessary in the light of contemporary obstetric knowledge and instruments. Presumably here Hamilton was proposing the use of forceps or craniotomy as these constituted the extent of obstetric knowledge and practice at that time.

6. Defective pelvis
Hamilton considered the degree of deficiency of space in the pelvis to be an important factor, but once again recommended the use of craniotomy rather than caesarean:

> 'Experience has proved, that where ready access is obtained for the admission of the necessary instruments, the head of the child may, by the operation of embryotomy, be so diminished... [that] the extraction of the mangled infant is practicable.' (pp. 270–71)

It appears from his writing that Hamilton had little regard for the discomfort and suffering of the pregnant woman, or for that matter, her child. But rather, he viewed them as interesting cases, useful only in terms of study and examination to enable him to analyse and theorize about the bodily functioning of womankind and nature itself. He recounted in great detail particular cases, charting every stage of complicated labours, including one case of a woman with extreme contraction of the pelvis where the pelvic gap was so narrow that Hamilton's instruments could not be introduced into the uterus in order to extract the child. Hamilton described the conditions of the woman from initial signs of labour, through extreme pain and vomiting, to the rupture of her uterus, and inevitably her death after many days of suffering. Undeterred by this, Hamilton went on to state:

> 'the histories of the operation, hitherto on record, do not appear to me to contain the ample information which would be required by one compelled to perform it.' (p. 293)

This is not surprising considering that the mortality rate from caesarean section in the early nineteenth century was 95 per cent (Routh, 1911). Thus British obstetricians were reluctant to perform the operation preferring instead to extract the infant through the natural passages by any means available. This would entail the use of forceps where possible, but in cases where the pelvic opening was too narrow the physicians would resort to the destruction of the infant (embryotomy or craniotomy) in order to extract it piece by piece. Hare (1838) was critical of the French and German surgeons who he said had boasted of their success with the caesarean operation and went on to praise British practitioners for not resorting to it: 'How thankful, then, ought we to be that scientific men have now invented instruments with the humane intention, if possible, of utterly eradicating this cruel operation' (p. 702).

The 'instruments' he referred to were the ones designed to destroy the infant. Regarding the caesarean section he went on to state: 'I sincerely trust that we may never again hear of its performance in this fair isle' (p. 702).

Even so, it was not the anti-caesareanists that deterred British obstetricians from performing the operation but rather the high mortality rate that continued to accompany it. In a series of lectures published in *The Lancet* in 1856, W. Tyler Smith said that the caesarean section should never be resorted to 'save in the utmost necessity' as the 'mother is almost surely sacrificed'. He went on to say: 'it is, and probably will ever remain, the most formidable operation which can be performed on the living body'. On the question of the circumstances under which the caesarean operation might be justifiable or even necessary, Tyler Smith stated that no point of importance in midwifery had been more keenly debated and less definitely settled at that time (p. 639).

Maternal mortality

One of the most detailed pieces of research into maternal mortality from caesarean section was that of Kayser of Copenhagen from 1750–1839. He suggested that there were many cases that were not reported, but that of 339 operations on record only 38 per cent of women survived. He felt this was an overestimate because in the 67 cases in which the operation was carried out in a hospital, where concealment would be much more difficult, the success rate was less at 20 per cent and he believed care would have been better than average (Tyler Smith, 1856). Kayser may have been wrong of course because infections were likely to be much more common in hospitals. However, one of his findings was that the success rate was improving. During the period 1750 to 1800 one third of women survived (32 per cent), from 1801–1832, 37 per cent survived, and from 1833–39 over half (51 per cent) lived. He also found that where the woman had been in labour seventy two hours or more, the success rate was only 28 per cent, while if labour was under 24 hours the success rate was four out of five (80 per cent) (Young, 1944).

The caesarean section was much more popular in the rest of Europe than in Britain during the eighteenth and nineteenth centuries despite the poor record in terms of patient survival. It appears that it was also safer. Much statistical evidence was optimistically presented to support or contend the practice of the caesarean section. Despite the dubious reliability of some of the data collected at that time, one thing was certain – caesarean section in Britain constituted a much more dangerous operation than in the rest of Europe and also, by that time, in the United States (see Table 3.1).

Period	United Kingdom			Other countries			Source
	Country	*n*	Survival rate	Country	*n*	Survival rate	
1750–1856	GB	63	29%	'Foreign'	321	46%	Churchill, 1856 i
to 1856	England	26	8%				Merriman, 1856 i
to 1862	Britain	–	14%				Murphy, 1862 ii
to 1865	GB & Ireland	77	14%				Radford, 1865
to 1866	UK	–	11%				Routh, 1911
to 1872				France	344	45%	Schroeder, 1873 iii
to 1872				Germany	712	47%	Schroeder, 1873 iii
to 1876	UK	–	16%				Routh, 1911
to 1877				USA	80	48%	Harris, 1874 ii
to 1879	GB	131	18%				Radford, 1880 iii
1852–1880				USA	120	42%	Young, 1944

(i from Tyler Smith, 1956; ii from Newell, 1921; iii from Francome et al.,1993)

Table 3.1: Some international rates of maternal survival from caesarean section in the nineteenth century

Many of the cases contained in the data given in Table 3.1 are likely to have been repeated in more than one of the collections. Further, the smaller sample sizes for the United Kingdom data may give a less favourable picture of the operation in those areas. It is also the case that all statistics are likely to present a more favourable picture of the operation than the real results as successful cases were reported more than the failures. However, the data could be interpreted as representing a small but gradual improvement in success rates towards the end of the nineteenth century, particularly in the United Kingdom. What these data do serve to highlight is the very high maternal mortality rate from the caesarean operation in general and the striking difference in success rates between the United Kingdom and the Continent in particular. Even so, in the words of W. Tyler Smith in 1856, 'The most favourable of these results are sufficiently discouraging' (p. 639).

Of course many explanations were forwarded for this anomaly between the United Kingdom and the rest of Europe including high alcohol consumption among British women and climatic differences (Young, 1944). It is more likely, however, to be due to the fact that on the continent the operation was performed on healthy women, the subjects of deformity, at the commencement of labour whilst the unwillingness on the part of the British practitioners to perform the caesarean section will have meant that the patients were already in a much weakened state by the time the operation was deemed to be necessary. It was often resorted to only after other means of delivery had failed. This coupled with the inexperience of the British in the operative technique meant that the prognosis would not have been good for women in the United Kingdom.

Religion would also have had a role to play in the discrepancy between the United Kingdom and the rest of Europe. The greater influence of the Church in Roman Catholic countries of Europe, with their emphasis on preserving the life of the child, or at least extracting the child in order that it may be baptized, would have rendered other techniques such as craniotomy obsolete, and explains, in part, the higher caesarean section rate in those countries. However, this does not mean that the caesarean operation was a completely safe endeavour in the rest of Europe. Catastrophic maternal mortality rates, mainly from infection which accompanied the technique, continued to be associated with caesareans. A German obstetrician, Osiander, is reputed to have said in 1805:

> 'One should allow the patient to draw up her will and grant her time to prepare herself for death before the operation.' (Allison, 1987, p. 546)

It appears that a difference in success rates was also found between those operations carried out in cities and those performed in rural areas. Tyler Smith (1856) believed that the operation had 'never been performed successfully in this metropolis' (London). He stated that: 'In the great capitals, London, Paris and Vienna, the mortality is far greater than in other places' (p. 639).

He may have been correct. Budin (1876) recorded a mortality rate of 100 per cent in Paris, that is, no successful caesareans performed between 1787 and 1875. Spath (1877) reported similar findings in Vienna (Newell, 1921). Tyler Smith's explanation for this anomaly between town and country was differences in the quality of the air: 'it is probable that a good air does more than the most skillful surgery' (1856, p. 641).

However a more plausible explanation is that women in the cities were more likely to be operated on in hospitals where, at that time, it was a more risky endeavour due to the fact that instruments were not sterilized and antiseptic principles were not strictly adhered to. Consequently mortality rates following caesareans were much higher in the hospitals at that time.

Infant mortality

It has been suggested that the caesarean section was resorted to for the safety of the child more frequently than for that of the mother (Tyler Smith, 1856). Historically this is certainly the case when considering early civilizations' emphasis on post-mortem caesareans and the Catholic Church's dictum of sacrificing the mother in order to baptize the child. However, Tyler Smith (1856) suggested that the performing of the operation in the hope of saving the child was misguided as 'the statistics of the operation demonstrate beyond question that the amount of fetal is almost equal to that of the maternal mortality' (p. 639). Yet the data quoted by Tyler Smith, while not demonstrating a good prognosis for the infant, did not support this argument as Table 3.2 demonstrates.

From the 77 cases recorded by Radford (1865), where the maternal mortality was 86 per cent, 78 infants were extracted (including one case of twins), 46 (59 per cent) of the infants survived and 32 (41 per cent) died. So it seems that the outcome of the caesarean operation was, on the whole, more favourable for the infant than it was for the mother. Radford claimed that nearly all the infants that did not survive were dead before the operation and it was his opinion that more infants might have been saved if the caesarean section had been performed earlier.

Maternal Mortality	Infant Mortality	Source
71%	46%	Churchill *
92%	57%	Merriman *

* from Tyler Smith, 1856

Table 3.2: Maternal and infant mortality from caesarean section by the mid 1800s

A royal catastrophe
The event of a royal birth in 1817 appears to have unwittingly furthered the cause of caesarean section in this country. Sir Richard Croft attending the labour of Princess Charlotte allowed an obstructed labour to continue in preference to using forceps or dismembering the heir to the throne of England. Fearing the death of the Princess from a caesarean section, Sir Richard did nothing. The infant was stillborn, the Princess died, and three months later Sir Richard shot himself (NIH, 1981). These events had major historical impact, apart from bringing Queen Victoria to the throne, marking an important turning point away from 'ultra-conservatism' in obstetrics, and could be seen by the more sceptical as a justification for the attitude 'when in doubt – operate!'.

The debate over caesareans in Britain and France
The British obstetricians were often critical of their European counterparts for carrying out caesareans unnecessarily. A French doctor in 1829 commented that when the smallest diameter of the pelvis was nearly two inches the child must be alive and the decision had to be taken whether to follow the English and destroy the infant or rather to give it life while exposing the mother to great danger. The French generally took the latter position while one English commentator said 'pity the poor French women we say' (Young, 1944, p.74). However, it would be wrong to assume that the French doctors never performed embryotomy, for in 1849 several cases were reported where it was tried before a caesarean was carried out (Young, 1944). The British obstetricians were much more conservative in their estimations of pelvic contraction that would indicate the necessity for the caesarean operation than their European counterparts. However, reports of the exact degree of pelvic deformity which would indicate a caesarean to British obstetricians varied considerably. After reviewing the evidence from 1822 to 1862 Young (1944) commented:

> 'The highest authorities in Great Britain at this time fixed the degree of pelvic contraction in which the dimensions varied from 3–3½ inches in the long diameter as the lowest limit below which delivery by embryotomy could be performed, and below which it was always necessary to perform a caesarean.' (Young, 1944, p. 76)

This estimation puts the British practitioners more in line with their counterparts in the rest of Europe. Reports from other sources demonstrate a much more restricted practice among the British. Churchill (1856) suggested that only when the antero-posterior diameter of the brim was not more than one inch was there no recourse but the caesarean operation. A Dr Rigby considered the operation unavoidable only when the child could not be extracted 'piecemeal' (sic) through the natural passages but did not give any positive measurements which would justify the operation in his opinion (Tyler Smith, 1856, p. 640).

The debate takes off in Britain

By the mid 1850s an important debate had begun among British obstetricians over the propriety of performing the caesarean operation in the light of the extremely high maternal mortality rate associated with the procedure. In order to open the discussion on the causes of failure of the operation and to ascertain whether it was possible to improve the outcome for the mother, Dr Charles West reported a case at a meeting of the Royal Medical and Chirurgical Society on 28th January, 1851. The case included details of a caesarean operation from which the patient did not fully recover and died four days later. Dr West reported a maternal mortality rate from the operation of 63 per cent from recorded cases since 1750 but went on to estimate that the rate should in fact be much higher as maternal mortality rates from caesarean carried out in hospitals in this country were 85.4 per cent or 87.5 per cent and that abroad they were 79 per cent (The Lancet, 1851a). Dr West went on to report only five successful cases of caesarean section in Great Britain since 1821 (The Lancet, 1851b).

Dr West's speech aroused great controversy within the Society. A response to it from Dr Robert Lee provided a good example of opinion among British Obstetricians at that time. Dr Lee quoted from Mauriceau (1681) when he said that there were very few, if any, cases of difficult labour, in which an experienced accoucheur would fail to extract the child, dead or alive, whole or in pieces, without resorting to the caesarean operation. Agreeing with this view, Dr Lee stated that he had never met a case of distortion of the pelvis, however great, where he had not succeeded in completing the delivery with the perforator and crochet (The Lancet, 1851a), highlighting the British tendency to favour modes of delivery that were destructive to the infant. However, Dr Lee's contention was that induction of premature labour was preferable to caesarean section saying that:

> 'It is altogether unaccountable that 39 years should have passed away after the safety, efficacy, and morality of inducing premature labour should have been demonstrated, that the practice should have remained almost unnoticed.' (The Lancet, 1851a)

Dr Lee continued to say that if in all cases of distortion of the pelvis, premature labour were induced at about the mid period of pregnancy, or as late as the sixth month, the caesarean operation would never be necessary. His opposition to the operation was based on his contention that in British midwifery no single well-authenticated instance was on record of a mother recovering after the performing of a caesarean operation (The Lancet, 1851a). Being totally opposed to the operation he stated:

'This rage for cruel and bloody operation has spread far and wide, and attempts are being made on all sides of this country, at the present moment, to pervert and corrupt the sound and fundamental doctrines of English midwifery. My conscience will not permit me to remain a silent witness of such abominations.' (The Lancet, 1851a)

In closing his speech, Dr Lee recounted the case of a woman in Cupar (Fife) who in 1847 'escaped from the horrors of the caesarean operation'. The patient was a 34 year old woman with great distortion of the pelvis. It was decided by Dr Simpson and three other practitioners that a caesarean section would be necessary. When labour commenced, Dr Simpson was called from Edinburgh, some 30 miles away. But on arriving in Cupar, he reported that he and his colleagues 'were surprised to hear that the patient was delivered, and our surprise was only increased by learning that no kind of instrumental aid had been required'. On announcing this at the meeting, Dr Lee sat down 'amidst the enthusiastic cheers of the Society, and loud roars of laughter from all sides' (The Lancet, 1851a, p. 155).

The debate was adjourned until February 11th, 1851, at which time the Society experienced one of its most crowded meetings with many members being turned away because of lack of space. At the meeting, Dr Murphy took exception to Dr Lee's speech the previous month, and protested against the principle of personal attacks which he felt had been demonstrated so enthusiastically at the end of the last meeting. He went on to state that Dr Lee's account of the caesarean proposed by Dr Simpson had not contained the full facts. The woman in question suffered from severe deformity of the pelvis and could not have delivered normally but for the fact that the child had been dead for some time in utero and was only able to pass through the pelvic opening because of its rather fluid and decomposed state (The Lancet, 1851b). Dr Murphy went on to reiterate West's original question and redirect the attention of the Society to the possibility of improving the outcome of caesarean section for the mother (The Lancet, 1851b). However, it appears that British practitioners were determined not to entertain such a discussion based on the assumption that the outcome for the mother was usually disastrous and destruction of the child as an attempt to save the mother preferable in most cases. Dr Ashwell insisted that:

'premature labour,... craniotomy, and the dismemberment of the child, with all their difficulty and delay, were far preferable to delivery by the Caesarean section.' (The Lancet, 1851b, p. 207)

British pro-caesareanists

Although in a notable minority, supporters of caesarean section were to be found among the obstetricians in nineteenth century Britain. G.S. Bedford (1844) and Thomas Radford (1865), who became one of the champions of caesarean section by highlighting the barbarous nature of craniotomy, were two such examples. Radford was one of the most influential commentators on caesarean section during that time. He wrote:

'To my knowledge, there has been no subject connected with medicine which has created more bitterness of feeling and animosity.' (p. 1)

In his book *Observations on the Caesarean Section and on Other Obstetric Operations*, Radford recommended the caesarean section for cases of contracted pelvis and also for blockage, for example, by certain types of tumour that are not movable. He believed that:

'The risk to infants in Caesarean births is not much greater than that which is contingent on natural labours, provided correct principles of practice are adopted.' (p. 8)

Regarding the high maternal mortality rate which accompanied caesarean section, Radford pointed to the unfavourable constitutional state of women prior to the operation and therefore recommended the performance of all obstetric operations, especially caesarean section, early in labour, stating that the danger from the operation increased with the duration of the labour. Similarly, Radford pointed out that the duration of labour exercised very great influence upon the condition of the infant, particularly after the membranes had ruptured. Thus:

'the deaths of the infants which have occurred in Caesarean cases are generally to be attributed to the long continued and violent pressure which they have endured during labour.' (p. 17)

However, Radford did point out that another cause of infant death, which was related to the caesarean operation specifically, was the seizure of the neck of the infant during extraction through the incised opening of the uterus.

In defence of the caesarean operation Radford proposed that obstetricians who performed the operation were simply imitating nature. He went on to say that when the usual passage is blocked, the 'natural' solution is the yielding of the uterine tissue thus making an opening for the escape of the fetus. This is followed by the ulceration in the abdomen whereby part after part of the infant passes through the opening, until the whole contents of the cyst are discharged – an extremely slow and hazardous process. Thus the caesarean operation is merely an imitation of nature although by a much more 'safe and an expeditious plan'. On the subject of post-mortem caesareans, Radford stated that they were necessary in order to do justice to the infant which was likely to be alive (p. 18).

It was the influence of Radford among the medical profession that began the shift in position towards a more accepting climate for the caesarean operation. Even so, for late nineteenth century Britain, the caesarean section continued to be a fatal operation and therefore only performed occasionally on a living woman, usually when craniotomy could not be performed, possibly because ovarian cysts prevented access to the infant. In other words, it would only be performed when everything else had been tried and failed (Newell, 1921). It is not surprising therefore that the first successful caesarean operations to be carried out in hospitals in the Western world did not occur until the end of the nineteenth century. The first one was performed in Dublin's Rotunda Hospital in 1889, followed by Boston's Lying-In Hospital in 1894, then the Saint-Antoine Hospital in Paris in 1896 and finally the Lille Charite Hospital in 1897 (Shorter, 1982).

The rest of the world?

Given the ethnocentricity of historical data, information relating to the performance of the operation in, for example, the third world, is scarce to say the least. However, the operation is recorded to have been performed at Katura, Uganda, in 1879. This event constitutes the first suggestion of the early development of the caesarean section by what were considered to be 'uncivilized' people. Robert W. Felkin (1884), a medical missionary, who was present for the surgery, described what he saw in great detail with illustrations. The patient was a twenty year old primiparous woman. Felkin noted that before the operation the practitioner anaesthetized the patient with banana wine which he then used to cleanse his hands and the patient's abdomen, thus displaying considerably more knowledge of asepsis than his so-called 'civilized' counterparts who only saw fit to wash their hands after the operation had been performed. The patient was tied to the bed for the operation which Bishop (1960) related thus:

> 'After first pronouncing an incantation he (the surgeon) gave a shrill yell and then made a quick incision, cutting through the abdomen and through the wall of the uterus. Bleeding points were touched by an assistant with a red-hot iron. The child was taken out quickly and handed over to an assistant. The cord was cut and the after-birth was removed by hand. The womb was not sutured, but the abdominal wound was covered temporarily with a porous grass mat, and the patient was raised to let the fluid out. Then the wound was closed with seven thin nails and string, very much as a chicken is trussed with skewers and string. The child was alive and the mother made a perfect recovery, her wound being healed on the eleventh day.' (Bishop, 1960, p. 27)

The skill and competence with which the operation in Katura was performed, and the precision with which every step of the operation was carefully planned in advance, suggests that the technique had been under development for a long time and therefore had been practiced by 'uncivilized' races with success, possibly for centuries, while it remained a most fatal, last resort, operation among 'civilized' nations.

CHAPTER FOUR

Caesarean Versus Other Techniques

At various stages throughout the history of obstetrics, different procedures, treatments, instruments and operations have been invented and tested to aid the delivery of the infant in difficult cases. While all attempts had one objective, to save the mother, child or both, they have at times been presented as preferable to the caesarean section and have affected the history of the operation in some way. During the eighteenth century surgeons began to experiment with other forms of surgical intervention to aid labour.

Caesarean versus symphyseotomy

In 1777, the poor success rate of the caesarean operation meant that it was almost entirely superseded by the development of a new operative delivery technique. The operation 'symphyseotomy' was introduced by a French surgeon, M. Sigault. His earliest proposal for the operation, suggesting that it should be tested on animals and condemned criminals, was not favourably received. The later proposal, which was successfully tested on a patient, consisted of cutting through the skin in the direction of the pubic bone and then dividing the junction of the cartilaginous symphysis with the knife. The knees of the patient which were being held firmly by assistants were then gently forced apart in order to separate the bones, thus making room for the delivery of the child under the strength of the uterine contractions. At the time, it seemed like a good idea.

> 'The section of the symphysis pubis, it was thought, would banish for ever the use of crotchets, of perforators and other destructive instruments, as well as premature delivery and the cesarean operation.' (Baudelocque, 1801, pp. 48–9)

Subsequent to his initial attempt, Sigault operated on four other women, one of whom died. Although Sigault was the first to propose and successfully perform the operation it was M. Le Roy, an assistant at the operation, who was the first to publish an account of it. However, opposition to the operation was strong. In 1803, Hamilton wrote:

> '... from the history of between 30 and 40 cases, where the division of the symphysis pubis was performed on the continent, and one case in Great Britain, we consider ourselves authorised to condemn that operation in every view, and advise that it be had recourse to *in no case whatever.*' (p. 333, original emphasis)

Up to 1830 there had been 41 symphyseotomies with 14 maternal and 28 fetal deaths, a maternal mortality considerably less than that of caesarean section at that time (Routh, 1911). However, as time went on, Sigault became less confident about the procedure and before his death he recommended caesarean section instead of symphyseotomy for cases of contracted pelvis (Young, 1944). Early commentators have suggested that the use of the symphyseotomy fell into disrepute allowing the use of the caesarean section to flourish (Newell, 1921).

This is not to say that symphyseotomy is no longer practiced. The procedure has been modified somewhat with the suggestion that if the incision is made during labour, the mere pressure of the baby's head will divide the two parts of the symphysis resulting in more space in the pelvis and a vaginal delivery, rather than the bones being forced to separate by assistants pressing apart the legs of the woman (Engelkes and van Roosmalen, 1992). Similarly, one of the main reasons why the operation was denounced as 'obsolete' was because of associated complications, such as risk of damage to the urethra. It has been suggested that this can now be prevented by the pre-operative insertion of a urinary catheter and the moving of the catheter to the side while the incision in the symphysis is made (Engelkes and van Roosmalen, 1992).

As recently as 1992 the symphyseotomy was recommended as preferable to caesarean section, particularly in certain cultures where failure to deliver vaginally may lead to stigmatization (Engelkes and van Roosmalen, 1992). The operation continues to be used in some countries and the Maternity Report of St. Lukes Hospital, Anua, Nigeria, revealed that in 1991 a total of 20 symphyseotomy operations were carried out (Francome et al., 1993). It has further been proposed that in some cases of obstructed labour due to cephalopelvic disproportion (CPD), symphyseotomy is a valuable substitute for caesarean section, as there is less mutilation, ultimately it obtains the same, or even faster, result, and often prevents a subsequent obstructed labour. The suggestion is that if safe precautions are taken, such as the insertion of a urethral catheter and pelvic fixation during and immediately after delivery to prevent orthopaedic disorders leading to serious walking problems, complications are minimal. Chances of future safe deliveries are also improved as the pelvic aperture will have been permanently widened and there is no risk of future scar rupture (Engelkes and van Roosmalen, 1992).

Caesarean versus craniotomy

During the first half of the nineteenth century, caesarean section became more popular with a consequent rise in rates for most of Europe. Britain, however, remained slow to catch on, obstetricians preferring the techniques more destructive to the child, such as craniotomy, judging the caesarean section as unjustifiably putting the mother's life at risk. This is not surprising considering that the maternal mortality rate was 89 per cent in 1866 and 84 per cent in 1876. It was suggested that it was not preference for the destruction of the child that lead British obstetricians to rely on craniotomy but rather the lack of a viable alternative for cases of contracted pelvis (Routh, 1911).

The main bone of contention between British obstetricians and their European counterparts was the degree of pelvic contraction and much argument ensued over the actual degree of contraction that should indicate the necessity for caesarean section.

Thus the British obstetricians used craniotomy in preference to abdominal delivery for cases in which European practitioners would have performed a caesarean.

Craniotomy is a difficult process by which the head of the infant is crushed in the womb in order to make it small enough to pass through the vaginal canal. This caused many problems as may be seen by some of the recorded case histories. J. Hamilton, for example, described in 1840 how in a woman with the width at the brim of only 1.5 inches he performed a craniotomy at midnight. He started his efforts to extract the child at 9.30 the next morning but did not succeed until two o'clock in the afternoon. The woman recovered and Hamilton was 'carried home in a sedan chair exhausted' (Young, 1944, p. 77).

Craniotomy was performed by the use of a variety of instruments, for example, penknife, scissors, pincers and various types of hook, basically anything that was available to the practitioner at the time. If the head was not the part of the body presenting, then the operation was called an embryotomy. There was continuing debate about the rectitude of killing the about-to-be-born child. Many argued that it had no sensation of feeling or pain (Young, 1944). In 1838 Hare published a letter in *The Lancet* in which he brought to the attention of the medical profession an instrument called the 'Osteotomist' or 'Bone-Pliers' which he described as the combined principles of a punch and a pair of scissors. The instrument was designed for the purpose of breaking up the infant so that it could be delivered through the natural passages. Hare stated that the osteotomist was:

> 'a power by which any portion of the foetal skeleton presenting at the brim of a contracted pelvis may be broken down into small fragments of about half an inch in diameter, with the most perfect impunity to the tissues of the mother.' (p. 702)

Given the higher caesarean rate in the rest of Europe, it is not surprising that craniotomy was correspondingly less common there. In Britain the operation occurred once in 219 deliveries compared to once in 1,205 deliveries in France and was even more rare in Germany with one in 1,944 deliveries. It appears that almost any method was preferable to the British obstetricians of that time, rather than resorting to caesarean section, who viewed the actions of the European obstetricians as more barbaric than their own. However, it was a difficult procedure and the obstetrician had to gather all the pieces together to make sure that nothing had been left inside the woman. There were strong critics. Many opposed craniotomy because of the mortality rate that accompanied it. The editor of *The Lancet*, Thomas Wakley, said in 1838 that 'the operation of crushing the child's head and extracting the body piecemeal is as fatal a proceeding as the Caesarean operation itself' (1838, p. 703).

Churchill, in 1842, gave the maternal mortality from craniotomy as about one in five. To make a comparison he collected data for 321 operations since 1750 and said that the majority of women (172) died. However, even such analysis did not undermine the essential fact that at the time maternal mortality was lower for craniotomy than caesarean section which in Britain was over 80 per cent (Routh, 1911). Such results were deemed to justify the position of the British obstetricians.

Despite the dominant British view being in favour of craniotomy there were a few in Britain who also became concerned with the loss of fetal life. In recounting the case of a caesarean that he had performed due to a contracted pelvis, where it was evident that the head of the infant could not pass through the pelvic opening, Vanderfuhr stated that he viewed craniotomy as a 'shocking resource'. He knew the child to be alive because he had felt its movements as had the mother and therefore saw no way forward but to perform a caesarean section (1826, p. 388). Bedford stated in 1844:

> 'The man who would wantonly thrust an instrument of death into the brain of a living foetus, would not scruple, under the mantle of night, to use the stilleto of the assassin.' (Young, 1944, p. 80)

In 1865 Radford calculated, on the evidence available to him, that 2,861 infants were being destroyed annually by this operation and suggested that this figure was an extremely conservative estimate. A determined opponent of craniotomy, Radford argued that if craniotomy was used certain great men (sic) would not have been born (an argument that was to be repeated later by opponents of birth control): 'Suppose the head of Shakespeare had been opened, what would have been the loss to society?' (p. 48). In addition he commented: 'It is one thing to deliver the woman, and another to do so safely. It is much to be deplored, that this operation is still permitted to be so unconditionally performed' (p. 48).

Many commentators objected to the use of craniotomy when the fetus was living and viable. Routh stated in 1911 that:

> 'as craniotomy necessarily involves foetal death, it is to be hoped that the time is not far distant when the increasing safety of Caesarean section will lead to its abolition when the child is alive.' (p. 8)

In Catholic countries the fetus was often given a very high status among theologians which meant that craniotomy could not be recommended. However, the views of opponents of craniotomy, including eminent physicians such as Radford and authorities such as the Catholic Church, did not hold much appeal among the medical fraternity, and the clear view among British obstetricians was that craniotomy was preferable, as the caesarean was such a dangerous operation that it must only be a last resort.

Caesarean versus forceps

Forceps, or 'high forceps' as they were known at the time, were in popular use as an aid to difficult deliveries during the nineteenth century. Once again there were proponents on both sides of the debate. For example, Radford (1865) claimed that:

> 'This instrument most justly takes a high position in obstetricy, because its sole employment is for the preservation of life. It is intended, within a certain range of protracted labour, to supersede craniotomy. In the hands of a discreet and judicious practitioner, it is both a safe and a very powerful instrument. Before its introduction into practice, whenever turning could not be performed, the child was doomed to destruction by craniotomy.' (p. 27)

Further, Radford stated that:

> 'There are no statistics published which afford any truthful information either as
> to the frequency of the application of this instrument, or as to the mortality of
> those women who have been delivered by it.' (p. 29)

He claimed that he had used forceps many times and never had a death as a result of
their application.

The superiority of forceps over craniotomy being established, the debate over the
relative benefits of forceps as opposed to caesarean section continued. In 1879, Harold
Williams attempted to prove statistically that delivery by forceps was much more
dangerous in terms of fatality to the mother than caesarean section (Young, 1944).
However, doubts remained and the debate over the relative benefits of forceps as
opposed to caesarean section still continues. The latest evidence shows that the use of
forceps has diminished as caesareans have become safer (Francome, 1990).

Caesarean versus induction

Induction of premature labour has been called an 'essentially British procedure' (Routh,
1911, p. 3). In 1756 a consultation of London obstetricians established it as the ethically
correct treatment for delivering cases of contracted pelvis. Over a hundred years later
Robert Barnes (1862) stated that:

> 'English Midwifery... claims the honour of introducing and establishing an
> operation which had probably been the means of saving more lives of mothers
> and children than any other operation we know of.' (Routh, 1911, p. 3)

In 1851 a Dr Lee argued in favour of induced labour over caesarean section saying that
he regarded it as the most important improvement ever introduced into the practice of
midwifery. He stressed that the value of induction of premature labour was that both
mother and child were preserved. He said that during the previous 55 years the operation
had been successfully performed in a great number of cases and the lives of many
children saved by it. Quoting statistics from his colleague, Dr H. Davies of Brighton,
who had performed the operation 50 times, he said that 29 children were born alive
and all mothers survived. Lee himself had performed the operation as many as 50
times with success including the case of one woman with a greatly distorted pelvis on
whom he had performed the procedure 12 times (The Lancet, 1851a).

Despite Lee's claims, Radford (1865) suggested that induction of premature labour
was never intended to supersede the caesarean section but, rather, to prevent
craniotomy. However, the induction of abortion was proposed for the purpose of
superseding the necessity of the caesarean section. According to Radford, in general,
by the time induction of labour was proposed, the woman had passed the period
when a caesarean could be advantageously performed. Radford objected to this situation
stating that induction was not as safe a technique as it was commonly presented, and
in some cases it had caused the death of the mother. Therefore, Radford advocated the

caesarean section instead. Yet by 1911, Routh still claimed induction of premature labour to be a 'favourite' method of dealing with cases of contracted pelvis in the United Kingdom.

Caesarean versus pelvitomia nova

Another alternative to the caesarean operation, the 'Pelvitomia nova' was suggested by John Aitken of Edinburgh in 1882. The aim of the operation was to make a segment of the pelvic girdle movable to allow delivery of the child in cases of extreme distortion or contraction of the pelvis. He tested this technique for the first time on a woman in Italy – both mother and child died (Young, 1944). Little reference has been made to the operation since that time.

CHAPTER FIVE

Self-Inflicted Caesareans

'Sisters were doing it for themselves'

Throughout history, many women have performed the caesarean operation on themselves. Although presumably unaware of surgical procedures, these operations were performed out of desperation. Most constituted attempts to conceal pregnancy and avoid the condemnation and ridicule that accompanied pregnancy outside of marriage in many cultures. In the majority of such cases the outcome was not good for the infant, often the child would die before or during the complicated labour, or the baby died due to mutilation from the surgery or suffocating in the amniotic fluid which would flood the abdomen during the operation.

The earliest known case of a woman performing the operation on herself was recorded to have occurred in 1769 in the West Indies. Mosely (1795) suggested that the woman had carried out the operation because of impatience (sic) with the pain of a prolonged labour (Baudelocque, 1801), although, of course, this explanation is that of the observer and not the woman herself.

On January 29th, 1822, a fourteen year old woman performed the operation on herself, constituting the first recorded case of such an event in the United States. The woman was carrying twins and delivered herself lying in a snow bank. On delivery of the first baby she buried it in the snow. Doctors were called in to remove the second child and to attend to the wound. The patient survived but the fate of the children is unknown (McClellen, 1822, in Young, 1944), although considering the conditions of the birth it is unlikely that either child lived.

In 1876, a woman in labour for three days performed a caesarean section, which she had heard was possible, on herself to obtain relief from abdominal distension and violent pain. The child did not survive, although it is possible that it was dead before the operation as the woman reported that fetal movements had ceased. Her wound was treated by a physician and she made a full recovery (Von Guggenburg, 1876, in Young, 1944).

In Turkey, in 1879, a woman cut open her abdomen and uterus with a razor after being in labour for over 36 hours and not progressing. The wound was then sewn up by a neighbour and both mother and child apparently survived (Young, 1944).

Madigan (1884) reported a case of a woman who cut open her abdomen and uterus with a razor and delivered a male child. According to Madigan, neighbours who found her with the placenta and dead child lying beside her were so frightened that they ran away. By the time the clergyman arrived the mother was also dead (Madigan, 1884, in Young, 1944).

In 1886, *The Lancet* recorded the case of a 23 year old single woman, seven months pregnant, who was talked about and faced a great deal of questioning from her family as to the reasons for her increase in weight. Fearing the shame which accompanied the bearing of an illegitimate child in Italy at that time, she cut open her abdomen with a sharp carving knife and brought out the baby in pieces. In the evening she took a cloth soaked in blood the few miles to her sister's house to 'prove' she had menstruated. Her subsequent illness led to medical attention and the operation being recorded in the medical records. Editors of *The Lancet* wrote to the doctors involved in the case and received confirmation and further details (Baliva and Serpieri, 1886).

From the limited evidence available on self-inflicted caesareans, it appears that women 'doing it for themselves' in history was actually safer than the so-called 'professional' procedures. An American medical historian, Harris, wrote in 1879 that a woman in labour had a 50 per cent chance of surviving a caesarean operation if she performed it herself compared to a 10 per cent reported survival rate if attended to by a New York surgeon. This is quite possible considering that the woman at home was more likely than the hospital surgeon to be using clean implements and was less likely to be using equipment that has just been used to carry out a postmortem or to perform surgery on a patient with a fatal infection. Harris later recorded a 66 per cent survival and recovery rate for women performing the operation on themselves compared to a rate of 37.5 per cent for American physicians up to 1888, and 14 per cent for their British counterparts (Harris, 1888).

This phenomena is not entirely unknown in the twentieth century. In 1901 a woman at full term in her fifteenth pregnancy is said to have self-performed the operation believing herself to be about to die from tuberculosis. Her wound was sewn by her thirteen year old daughter and both mother and child recovered. Further, a woman is reputed to have admitted herself to hospital in 1913 with an abdominal wound which was found to contain remnants of placenta. The child had apparently been allowed to drop into a bucket of water in which it drowned. The woman recovered (Young, 1944).

CHAPTER SIX

Development of the Operative Technique

Despite improvements in the operative technique for caesarean section in the early nineteenth century, it was not until around the 1880s that the surgical technique for the operation began to be reviewed and defined, mainly by German doctors. Before that time the exact technique of each operation could have been as individual as the surgeons performing them. For example, in 1805 a German obstetrician, Osiander, devised a caesarean operation which involved keeping a hand in the vagina during the abdominal extraction of the infant (Allison, 1987). However, the increasing documentation of the most successful techniques, coupled with the invention of chloroform anaesthesia by Simpson of Edinburgh in 1847 and the ratification of antiseptic principles in surgery in 1867 by Lord Lister, meant that caesarean section became a more feasible option.

However, as highlighted previously, this option was not taken up immediately. Other emergency approaches such as forceps, craniotomy or symphyseotomy were used in preference to the caesarean. This is not surprising considering that the caesarean section operation during the nineteenth century continued to carry an extremely high maternal mortality rate. Radford (1865) stated that: 'The statistics of the results of the caesarean section, especially as concerns the mothers, are highly unfavourable' (p. 7). One of the greatest risks to women from the caesarean operation during the nineteenth century was haemorrhage or infection. 'In many cases no attempt at repair or the formation of new tissue takes place; in others actual sloughing and loss of substance occurs, the wound gaping widely' (Tyler Smith, 1856, p. 639).

The procedure for caesareans

In a series of lectures which appeared in *The Lancet* in 1856, W. Tyler Smith gave details of the procedure for the caesarean section:

> 'The temperature of the room should be raised, with a view to the prevention of peritonitis, and chloroform administered, unless some special contra-indication exists. The abdominal incision may be made in the direction of the linea alba, or it may be oblique or horizontal, according as the configuration of the abdomen is altered by deformity. The situation of the placental attachment should be avoided, if this organ be attached anteriorly. This may be learnt by auscultation

before the operation is commenced. Great care is required in opening the peritoneum, so as to avoid wounding the intestines. The abdominal incision should be from eight to ten inches in length; and the uterine incision should be of nearly the same length. Some have advised that the liquor amnii should be evacuated before the commencement of the operation. When the amnion is punctured through by the uterine incision, care must be taken to let as little of the fluid as possible enter the peritoneal cavity. It is recommended to be removed carefully with pieces of sponge or a syringe. When this has been evacuated, the foetus is to be taken out, cautiously as in some cases the uterus has grasped the body or neck of the child at the wound, and rendered its extraction a matter of difficulty. The placenta is to be separated by the hand, and haemorrhage arrested by mechanical pressure, or the application of cold, the risk of peritoneal inflammation being the only objection to the latter. After the removal of the placenta, and the cessation of haemorrhage, all blood and fluid are to be carefully removed from the peritoneum, and the edges of the uterine and abdominal incisions brought together and maintained by sutures. The external wound is further to be dressed lightly with strapping and wet lint, and the whole supported by a many-tailed bandage, space being left for the exit of discharge. After the operation, large and continued doses of opium, with nutriment and stimulus in good quantity, appear to offer the best chances of recovery. Throughout, every care should be given to the avoidance of peritoneal irritation as far as possible; the escape of the bowels through the wound; and the suppression of haemorrhage.' (p. 641)

Thus by the mid 1850s, although some recognition of the risk of infection is evident, there was no reference to antiseptic principles such as the scrubbing of the physicians hands or sterilization of equipment to be used in the operation.

However the exact procedure for each operation continued to vary according to the surgeon performing the surgery. For example, it was not unknown for practitioners to suture the external wound in the early 1800s, while some later practitioners would suture the uterine wound only and close the external wound with bandages or sticking plaster. Others saw fit to leave both wounds gaping. There were similar anomalies in the use of anaesthesia. In 1826, Vanderfuhr recounted a case of a caesarean he had performed where, although no anaesthesia was used, 'during the whole operation the patient was perfectly tranquil; she did not utter a single cry'. But he did unite the wound with sutures, strips of adhesive plaster, dry lint, compresses and a bandage (p. 388). Mother and child apparently survived.

The 'Porro' operation

In 1876, Porro of Pavia recognized that the greatest risk to the patient was caused by haemorrhage from the incision in the uterine walls and from the escape of infected lochia into the peritoneal cavity. He therefore advised amputation of the body of the uterus in order to lessen the dangers of haemorrhage and infection; in other words, he used a sterilizing technique whereby a partially complete hysterectomy was performed after the caesarean birth. Porro carried out the first successful operation using his new method on 21st May 1876. The woman had been under observations for 24 days and the operation was carried out seven hours into labour. Porro and his assistants washed their hands in a dilute solution of carbolic acid and administered chloroform to anaesthetize the patient. The mother and child survived. This procedure was followed by such an improvement in the results of the operation that it soon became very popular (Newell, 1921). Despite the fact that Porro is usually credited with the discovery of this technique he was not, in fact, the first to use it. Storer of Boston had used amputation of the uterus on a case of multiple fibroids of the uterus in 1868 but apparently did not realize the importance of the innovation and credit therefore went to Porro for bringing the procedure to the attention of the medical world (Newell, 1921).

When others tried the operation the results at first were mixed. In fact the next three women to be operated on using the Porro method died, but two children lived. Three out of the first four women operated on in the United States died, and four out of the first five in Britain. However, some places showed a remarkable improvement and none greater than the Vienna Lying-In Hospital, where in the previous one hundred years not a single woman had recovered. From 1877 to 1885 there were 27 Porro operations with nearly half (48 per cent) of the women surviving. In the following three years there was a remarkable series of operations and out of 27 cases all except two of the women lived (Newell, 1921).

The first successful Porro operation to be performed in Britain was carried out by Dr Clement Godson in 1884. He recounted the case in the *British Medical Journal* (BMJ) and listed 137 operations by others with a maternal mortality rate of 55.8 per cent (Routh, 1911). Thus it was the Porro operation that was regularly adopted in England at that time. Harris (1888) advanced a number of reasons for the improved results of the Porro operation. These included:

- Carrying it out electively and not as a last resort.
- Operating early in labour.
- Rigid antisepsis.
- Washing all the blood out of the abdominal cavity.
- Antiseptic treatment of the stump (p. 150).

There was some opposition to the operation on the grounds that it sterilized the woman. One of the most vehement arguments appeared in the *American Journal of Obstetrics* (AJO) where Schlemmer (1883) argued that the operation was against religious tenets and that men should not have marital intercourse with wives who had undergone it. In contrast the English writer Playfair (1886) said that many women needing caesareans suffered from rickets and came from the poorer parts of the community suffering from ill nourishment. He continued to suggest the sterilization may have been of benefit to the community! Others prophetically saw Porro's method as a transitory one and this is in fact what it became.

The 'Sanger' method

The operation was revolutionized in 1882 by Max Sanger (1853–1903) who replaced the Porro technique with a process of closing the uterus in layers by the use of sutures or stitches. This was to:

> 'close the uterine wound by a system of deep (muscular) and superficial (peritoneal) sutures and so keep the uterine and peritoneal cavities shut off.' (The Lancet, 1891, p. 885)

Prior to this development the uterine incision was not usually sutured for fear of leaving suture material in the peritoneal cavity (Holland, 1921a). Sanger did not make any grand claims about having invented a new method of operating, rather he painstakingly studied the developments and innovations of the operation, comparing success rates, and came to a conclusion which brought together the best of what had gone before. For example, sutures had first been used by some practitioners in earlier times but it was not until Sanger published an article describing his technique in 1882 that they came into general use. This was an important development in the history of the caesarean section because it meant that hysterectomy was not necessary and, as such, it became known as the 'conservative' or 'classical' caesarean section as opposed to Porro's 'radical' operation (Newell, 1921).

The first operation following Sanger's recommendations was carried out by G. Leopold in Leipsig on 25th May, 1882, where the mother and child made a full recovery. However, the next two operations were not successful. It is surprising that Sanger himself did not carry out the operation according to his own suggestions until 4th December, 1884, when it was the tenth to be performed. Both mother and child made a good recovery.

Analysis of the first fifty Sanger operations up to 1887 showed that 70 per cent of women survived compared to only 40 per cent of the first fifty Porro operations (Harris, 1888). Closer analysis of the data showed that of the first 50 operations, 33 were done in Germany and all but one of the children and all but four of the mothers survived. However, of 17 operations carried out in other countries, only six mothers lived (Young, 1944). This may in part be because in Germany the criteria for performing the operation had been relaxed but is probably also indicative of greater experience and skill.

In February 1889 Dr Champneys of London drew attention to the value of Sanger's improved technique and described a successful case that he had performed in March 1888. In the next month, Dr Murdock Cameron of Glasgow had another successful case and in March 1891 he was able to publish a list of ten consecutive operations with maternal survival in nine cases. It has been said that Champneys' paper stemmed the tide which had been set in favour of Porro's radical operation towards a technique that was less mutilating for the mother (Routh, 1911).

The lower-segment operation

It was at the time when Sanger was publicizing his new technique that Kehrer first introduced the idea of using a lower uterine segment incision for the caesarean operation, believing it necessary to permit the safe closure of the uterine wound thereby reducing the risk of haemorrhaging and infection (Young, 1944). This important modification to the operative technique meant that the caesarean section became less of a dangerous endeavour than was previously the case. An indication of this was published in *The Lancet* (6 January, 1886). Dr Playfair referred to the statistics of caesareans published by the French obstetrician M. Dufeilley which showed that where the operation was performed in favourable circumstances, 80 per cent of women recovered compared to a success rate of 17 per cent in unfavourable conditions. He commented that these were better results than had been obtained in England, but went on to suggest that even the small success rate of 11 per cent was surprising considering 'the semi moribund condition in which the patients generally had been found before the operation'. However, he further concluded that the statistics 'at least prove that the caesarean section need not be the almost certainly mortal operation we were generally thought to consider it' (Playfair, 1886).

During the 1890s a liberalization of attitudes towards the operation occurred. An article based on a meeting appeared in *The Lancet* entitled 'Modern methods of caesarean section' in April 1891. This drew attention to the improvements in the operation brought about by Sanger whose results had originally been published in the United States in 1882 but were not reported in either *The Lancet* or the *BMJ*. The technique, however, was finally introduced in 1886 (The Lancet, 19 May 1894).

It seems that it was around 1890 that instruments began to be sterilized. Dr Lewers was reported in the *BMJ* in 1911 as saying: 'He could remember when generally the instruments were not boiled in surgical practice; this was not much more than 20 years ago, if, indeed, it was quite so long' (4 March).

In 1892 a meeting was reported in *The Lancet* where Dr Murdoch Cameron described his experience of performing caesareans. He had carried out fifteen, only two of the women had died and in neither case was their death due to the operation. Demonstrating that the lower segment incision was not in general use in Britain in the late nineteenth century, he described his procedure as follows:

> 'If labour has not set it should be induced, then a five or six inch incision in the abdominal wall ought to be made. The uterus is not brought out until the foetus has been extracted. Any rotation is carefully rectified, and a small incision made in the median line until the membranes (which must not be ruptured) are reached. Next the incision is enlarged upwards and downwards, and the child extracted. The uterus is now brought out and thoroughly emptied of placenta and membranes. The edges of the uterine incision are everted by an assistant and deep carbolised silk sutures inserted, with, if necessary a few cat gut ones.'
> (Cameron, 1892, p. 594)

Further developments in the operative technique

Frank of Cologne proposed a new operative method in 1907 – the transverse incision. By this method, under ideal conditions, the whole operation could be performed extraperitoneally therefore lessening the danger of peritoneal infection (Newell, 1921). However Newell stated that Frank's claim that his operation was safe, even when the conservative operation was absolutely contra-indicated, did not stand the test of time and thus the procedure proposed by Frank was continually modified and developed by other German surgeons, including Latzko and Sellheim. For example, in 1912 Kronig introduced a technique whereby peritoneal flaps were developed and the uterine segment closed vertically (Young, 1944). Similarly, Kustner reviewed the whole subject of caesarean section in 1915 and carefully reported his own modification to the technique based on his personal experience of 112 operations (Newell, 1921).

By 1919 Beck had further refined the caesarean operation and developed more subtle techniques. In 1921 he reported 83 operations performed using his moderated technique with a success rate of 96.4 per cent. While acknowledging certain technical difficulties, Beck was eager to point out the advantages of his method which included lessened susceptibility to haemorrhaging, a shorter recovery period and considerably reduced risk of uterine scar rupture in the event of subsequent pregnancies (Young, 1944).

Kehrer's lower segment operation (1882) was introduced into the United Kingdom in 1921 by Eardley Holland and Munro Kerr following dissatisfaction with the classical operation (Holland, 1921a). Holland highlighted what he considered to be the 'defects' of the classical operation: they were risk of sepsis in infected or suspected cases, risk of rupture of the scar, risk of intestinal complications during convalescence (although he did concede this to be a rare complication of the operation), and adhesions between the uterine scar and intestine, omentum or abdominal wall. According to Holland the advantages of the new method which avoided these 'defects' were the position of the wound which allowed better healing; less bleeding from the incision as it was made through a less vascular area; the ease of suturing as the edges of the wound are thin; no risk of adhesions to intestines, omentum or abdominal wall because of the position of the wound; less likelihood of infection; less disturbance to the abdominal contents and the fact that the scar was less likely to rupture during subsequent pregnancies and/or labour.

However, there was not total agreement over the propriety of the lower segment operation. Newell (1921) suggested that up until the time that he was writing it was Kustner's operation which seemed to hold out a greater promise of success than other modifications. He reported that at that time some authors, for example J.B. Delee (and presumably Holland and Kerr), were urging abandonment of the classical section in favour of the lower segment (or extraperitoneal) operation. Newell, however, felt that it was too early to pass judgement on their claims, although he did suggest that, in his experience, the classical operation performed on healthy women under ideal conditions had advantages over the extraperitoneal method and was a less difficult surgical procedure.

Better results

In 1926 Munro Kerr recorded four deaths from a reported 107 cases of the lower segment operation. However, British obstetricians were reluctant to adopt the new methods and it was not until 1931 when an article by J. St. George Wilson of Liverpool was published in which he reported 50 cases with only one death, that their attitudes began to change and the operation came into popular usage. Obstetricians became eager to publish the high success rates of their operations and a proliferation of statistics and articles followed, one of the most impressive being C. M. Marshall's report in 1939 of 245 cases without a single maternal death (Young, 1944).

The reduced risk of the operation as reflected in a steady decline in maternal mortality, from 12 per cent in the 1890s to 4 per cent by the 1930s (Young, 1944), produced not a decline in the rate of medical intervention in childbirth but rather a move away from the older style intervention techniques to a surgical procedure that appeared to be proving itself less damaging to the mother.

Medical indications for caesarean section in history

Today there are many reasons why caesarean sections are performed. Some indications have little to do with the pregnant woman or her baby and more to do with the organization or availability of hospital services (see Chapter 10). However, certain physiological conditions of pregnancy and labour continue to dominate as causal factors in caesarean section. Historically, the conditions leading to caesarean section have varied. It was not until 1604 that the physical condition of the woman prior to labour, namely the size of her pelvis, was deemed an important indicator for caesarean section. In 1798 one of the most comprehensive lists of circumstances which may necessitate the use of the operation was written. Most of the 'reasons' revolved around variations of the restricted pelvis and also included uterine rapture, abnormal presentation, deformity of the fetus and extra-uterine gestation (Hull, 1799). By 1801 the condition of tumours of the vagina had been added as an indication for caesarean section (Baudelocque, 1801).

Therefore during the nineteenth century the main indications for performing the caesarean operation were:

1.   Size of pelvis, for example, locked, contracted or deformed pelvis.
2.   Lacerated uterus.
3.   Ventral conception (fetus growing outside of the uterus).
4.   Uterine hernia.
5.   Position of the child, for example, breech presentation (Hamilton, 1803).

By the beginning of the twentieth century the main indicators for caesarean section had changed little, contraction and deformities of the pelvis generally being considered as absolute indications. There was a great deal of debate regarding the measurements pertaining to the exact degree of contraction. However, some commentators pointed out the futility of discussing absolute measurements of the pelvis without relating such dimensions to the size of the fetal head (Young, 1944).

For the mid-twentieth century Young (1944) also lists as indicators: pelvic tumours, cancer of the cervix, uterine haemorrhage, cardiac disease, dystocia, eclampsia, placenta praevia, breech and other abnormal presentations.

	Britain			USA	
n	182	436	256	140	573
	%	%	%	%	%
Contracted pelvis	74.0	62.3	63.0	47.0	57.0
Placenta praevia	6.0	8.0	12.0	6.0	7.5
Cardiac disease	7.0	9.4	7.4	4.3	3.6
Breech presentation	3.3	1.3	3.5	–	1.0
Pre-eclampsia	–	4.5	4.0	7.0	5.0
Eclampsia	(1 case)	0.4	1.2	1.7	2.4
Miscellaneous	9.3	12.9	8.6	34.0	23.3
Source	McIlory, 1932 *	Haultain et al., 1933 *	Kerr, 1937 *	Greenhill, 1931 *	Lull, 1933 *

* from Young, 1944

Table 6.1: Indications for caesarean section (early twentieth century)

By the mid twentieth century the main indications seem to have changed little, thus for the 1950s the conditions were: size of pelvis, placenta praevia and toxaemia. But by the 1960s other indicators had come to the fore such as poor obstetric history and placental insufficiency. By the 1970s the use of electronic fetal monitoring began to have an effect on the caesarean section rate and is reflected in the main indications for the operation: repeat caesareans, fetal distress, increased use of intrapartum fetal monitoring and breech presentation (Chalmers and Richards, 1977).

CHAPTER SEVEN

Caesareans in the Twentieth Century

By the end of the nineteenth century the improved operating conditions, including the use of antiseptic techniques and anaesthesia for pain, allowed greater latitude in choosing to use the caesarean section. The increased experience of surgeons in the procedure led to greater surgical competence bringing an improved post-operative success rate. The attitudes of medical practitioners to caesarean delivery began to change and the operation became more widely accepted.

'Once a caesarean, always a caesarean'?

It was in the early twentieth century that Edward Craigan made his famous pronouncement: 'Once a caesarean, always a caesarean' on 12th May 1916 (Hansell et al., 1990). At the time, this was not an unreasonable claim for two reasons. First, the main indicator for caesarean section during the nineteenth century and the early part of the twentieth century was cephalopelvic disproportion, usually due to deformity of the pelvis, thus the dictum would hold true as the indication for the original caesarean would be present in any subsequent pregnancies. Secondly, the use of the vertical incision, which was more prone to rupture than the lower segment incision introduced later, also meant that repeat caesareans were advisable.

However, Craigan's statement has been used to justify the practice of repeat caesarean for over eighty years, particularly in the United States. Yet this is, in fact, an erroneous interpretation of his original lecture. Craingan's aim was to promote conservatism in the use of the caesarean section. Concerned over the rising rates, he advised caution in performing the first caesarean as this would sentence a woman to a life-time of caesareans for subsequent pregnancies because 'once a caesarean, always a caesarean'. As the number of indications for caesarean section have increased significantly since the time that Craigan was lecturing and operative techniques have been substantially modified, including the use of the lower segment incision in almost all cases, the dictum is now outdated and obsolete.

Maternal mortality in the early twentieth century

By the beginning of the twentieth century it was possible to have good results with caesarean section unless women were operated on late in labour, had received repeated vaginal operations or been subject to other techniques, such as failed forceps or version. A major article appeared in the *Journal of Obstetrics and Gynaecology of the British Empire* in January 1911 by Dr Amand Routh. It drew attention to the different mortality as a result of the caesarean operation according to the condition of the woman. In favourable conditions it was 2.9 per cent but in suspect conditions it was 17.3 per cent. When the woman had been previously examined or attempts were made to deliver by other means the death rate was 34.3 per cent. The implication was that it was better to carry out the operation earlier rather than later, as Radford had suggested almost fifty years earlier.

Maternal death as a result of the caesarean operation began to decline, probably due to the advances in medical care such as improved anaesthetic techniques, blood products and blood transfusions, a wider variety of antibiotics for the treatment of infection, and better medical control of maternal illnesses such as diabetes, hypertension and heart disease. Routh (1911) recorded that the mortality rate from caesarean section had steadily diminished from 38 per cent in Glasgow between 1891–1900, to 20 per cent in 1902, and by 1904 it had reduced to 12 per cent. Moreover, he believed that in the United Kingdom the caesarean section was an operation with 'hardly any morbidity' (p. 16).

In 1921 Eardley Holland and Munro Kerr carried out the first comprehensive survey and audit of caesarean sections in order to ascertain the maternal mortality rate for the different indications. They gathered data for 4197 caesareans carried out in Great Britain and Ireland between 1911 and 1920. Eighty per cent were performed because of contracted pelves; 5.5 per cent for eclampsia and other toxaemias of pregnancy; 5 per cent for antepartum haemorrhage and the final 9.5 per cent for other conditions. They found that the maternal mortality rate for contracted pelves was 4.1 per cent but highlighted, once again, that the condition of the woman at the time of the operation had an effect on the outcome. The mortality rate among women operated on late in labour was 10 per cent and 27 per cent among cases operated on after attempts had been made to deliver with forceps or craniotomy (Holland, 1921b). The most likely explanation for the success of the operation for contracted pelves is that the condition could usually be ascertained before the onset of labour and therefore the operation performed early, which meant that the woman had a greater chance of survival.

Rising caesarean rates

Nonetheless, the British obstetricians of the early twentieth century were reluctant to switch to the new method of intervention, preferring instead their tried and trusted methods such as craniotomy. British obstetric textbooks continued to demonstrate this preference, while such destructive techniques had been rejected by practitioners in the United States and the rest of Europe. Early editions of *Williams Obstetrics* (1908) recommended the use of craniotomy instead of caesarean. However, the tide of change had begun in favour of abdominal delivery and by the 1930s and 1940s later editions of the book proposed the caesarean section and a more 'restricted' use of craniotomy

(Shorter, 1982). Some doctors clearly felt it was time for caesareans to replace destruction of the baby. In a discussion of the subject one doctor, Hastings Tweedy, said it was time that craniotomy on the living child was relegated 'to its place amongst the obsolete barbarities of the past' (BMJ, 4 March, 1911).

Therefore, from the beginning of the twentieth century, in terms of the use of the operation as a birthing technique, caesarean section had taken off. Although its transition into popular use was slow to begin with, in the 1930s caesarean section still remained less frequently used than forceps delivery and less often performed than vaginal delivery in cases of breech presentation, there was no looking back. Routh demonstrated the increase in use of caesareans in the case of Queen Charlotte's Hospital. From 1890 to 1899, out of 10,529 deliveries, only seven were carried out by caesarean. Between 1900–1909 there were 15,222 deliveries, an increase of 50 per cent, with caesareans increased ten fold to 74 by 1910. The main switch was away from craniotomy which declined from 28 per cent of births in the first decade to 13 per cent in the second (Routh, 1911). Between 1900 and 1909 one per cent of all births in the United States hospitals were by caesarean section. By the 1940s this figure had risen to three per cent. Britain's record was similar – in Dublin's Rotunda Hospital the rate for the caesarean operation was over two per cent by the 1940s (Shorter, 1982).

By the 1920s some discussion had begun on the long term effects of caesarean section. At this stage attention was concentrated on the outcome of subsequent pregnancies. In 1920 the *BMJ* reported a meeting at which Dr Eardley Holland gave details of 1,089 caesareans which had been followed up. Of these, 610 women had no further pregnancy, in part because sterilization was often performed at the same time. Of the 479 who had a subsequent pregnancy, 133 had abortions or miscarriages but there had been a total of 396 subsequent births with more than four out of five of them (82 per cent) being performed by caesarean (Young, 1944).

Indications for caesareans

The major focus of concern and the subject of much debate in the 1920s was the indications that would necessitate the performing of a caesarean operation. The changes in technique in the early part of the twentieth century meant there was continuous debate over what the indications for caesarean section should be. R.W. Holmes argued in 1915 that the operation had become a sort of 'makeshift' for real obstetric practice. He pointed out that those who were carrying out caesareans for reasons such as high blood pressure must accept the responsibility for deaths in subsequent pregnancies if the uterus ruptured. He argued that such deaths should be considered in calculating the mortality rates for first caesareans (Holmes, 1915).

J.T. Williams advocated that there should be a caesarean for all cases where there was breech presentation for a primiparous woman (Williams, 1916, in Young, 1944). In 1916 the *BMJ* published an article by R. Gordon Bell of Sunderland who detailed a successful caesarean he had performed on a woman with a contracted pelvis whose two previous pregnancies had ended in the destruction of the child in both cases (Bell, 1916). The same journal, however, carried a cautionary article by F.S. Kellogg entitled 'Caesarean section overdone'. In the following year Whitridge Williams (1917) told the Clinical Congress of Surgeons of the United States:

> 'Advances in the practice of medicine and surgery are rarely attained in a thoroughly rational manner, but that a period of undue enthusiasm, or even absurd reckless abuse, usually precedes the establishment of the actual value of a given procedure... I believe that we are at present going through such a stage in connection with Caesarean section.' (Young, 1944, p. 165)

In 1921 the *Journal of Obstetrics and Gynaecology of the British Empire* published an index to volume 28 dedicated to a discussion of caesarean section with contributions from prominent individuals in the contemporary medical fraternity. Munro Kerr's contribution was a discussion of the indications for caesarean section. The major indication at that time, he said, was contracted pelvis (84 per cent of cases), followed by tumours, eclampsia, placenta praevia, accidental haemorrhage and, to a lesser extent, ventralfixed uterus, interposition operation, prolapse of the cord, impacted shoulder presentation, abnormal conditions in the child, retraction and contraction rings, rigidity of cervix and vagina and grave diseases threatening the life of the mother. However, he summed up by stating:

> 'I am quite convinced that twenty years hence, when the youngest here have become the seniors, the accepted indications for Caesarean section will be extended even beyond the limits suggested.' (p. 348)

As the operation became safer (measured in terms of maternal mortality), following the introduction of the classical operation by Sanger in 1882, the indications for the operation began to steadily increase. However, the rapidly growing list of indications for the operation gave rise to a certain amount of concern, even among proponents of the caesarean such as Kerr and Holland. Holland stated that 'No operation has in modern times had its list of indications so widely, and as some consider so recklessly, extended as Caesarean section' (1921a, p. 349).

The anti-caesarean backlash

Not surprisingly opponents of the operation seized the opportunity to attack the widespread use of the caesarean. Blacker (1921) criticized Kerr and Holland for over-reliance on abdominal delivery. Whilst acknowledging the success of the operation on 'suitable cases' in 'suitable surroundings' in which proper asepsis could be assured, Blacker questioned the use of the operation for conditions where there was no proof of its success. He suggested that the increase in the number of operations being performed had led not to the precise definition of indications but rather to the widening of the number of indications. He concluded that when indications such as 'uterine inertia, epilepsy, hydramnios, varicose veins and abdominal pain' are recorded, the only explanation could be 'operative zeal of the practitioner' rather than 'knowledge and judgement' (p. 447).

Blacker compared Kerr and Holland's statistics for cases of contracted pelves which demonstrated a maternal mortality from caesarean section of 4.1 per cent, with data on the mortality rate of women with contracted pelves who had delivered spontaneously, which was less than one per cent (.09 per cent) (Blacker, 1921). His suggestion therefore was that even in cases of obvious contraction of the pelvis, it was still safer for the woman to be left to deliver spontaneously than being subjected to a caesarean section. His argument centred on the fact that whilst maternal mortality from caesarean section had been reduced significantly, there was still an element of risk involved and therefore the operation could not be resorted to as an easy option. Believing that the life of the mother should not be sacrificed in an attempt to save the life of the child, Blacker recommended craniotomy for cases where spontaneous delivery could not occur. The maternal mortality from craniotomy at that time was six per cent where the child was already dead and 1.3 per cent where the procedure was performed on a living child. Blacker therefore questioned the justification of performing the caesarean operation which involved a maternal mortality of four per cent at the best and 27 per cent at the worst. He said:

> 'No obstetrician undertakes such an operation as craniotomy on a living child without the greatest repugnance, but to pretend that this operation can be replaced without greater danger to the mother by such procedures as pubiotomy or Caesarean section, no matter how skillful the attendant, is to shut one's eyes to the truth.' (p. 454)

Caesarean sections: good use or abuse?

The debates of the early twentieth century marked an important turning point in medical attitude towards caesarean section and during 1921/22 the seeds were sewn for a new type of caution towards the operation. The suggestion was made that abdominal delivery could be abused. This position was not new. Almost 140 years earlier William Dease (1783) had suggested that the operation was being used to further the reputations of obstetricians rather than for medical necessity. What was new, however, was the contention that the operation could be abused for medical convenience. In 1922 the *BMJ* led with a major editorial on caesareans. It commented: 'No subject in obstetrics or gynaecology is being more talked about and discussed at present than caesarean section' (p. 277).

It stated that the increase in popularity was largely due to the collected statistics of Dr Routh in 1911. It went on to say that there was a danger that the operation could become a panacea for all obstetric ills and quoted Dr Blacker who had said that the ease and safety of the caesarean operation was leading to its abuse. It also drew attention to the accusation of Dr Franklin Newell, Professor of Clinical Obstetrics at Harvard, that the caesarean was the most abused obstetric operation:

> 'The operative indication has been a slow though normal labour which the attendant has hastened to end in the manner easiest for himself though often not best for the patient.' (p. 277)

The conclusion in the *BMJ* was that there was a temptation to perform an easy, quick and dramatic operation instead of following the safer and better, but more tedious, path of ordinary obstetric methods. It continued to argue that the increased number of indications for the operation 'is enough to show that the operation is indeed being abused here and now'. It went on to state that the view of one eminent and experienced obstetrician was that:

> 'The art and science of midwifery have either been lost by the younger generation in this country or will certainly be lost if this mad rage for caesarean section is continued.' (p. 278)

The editor conceded that the operation often led to a better outlook for the child, but agreeing with Blacker, argued that the profession should not lose its sense of the proportionate value of maternal life as compared to that of the infant. Stating that only in exceptional circumstances was it justified to expose the woman to increased risk in the interests of the 'unborn child' (p. 278).

Too many caesareans?

The debate over 'whether to section or not to section' which began among obstetricians in the sixteenth century continued into the early twentieth century (as it does today). This led to continual concern over the number of operations being performed. One very important contribution to the debate came from Plass, writing in the *American Journal of Obstetrics and Gynecology* in 1931. His argument was based upon the fact that there was still a significant maternal mortality rate associated with the caesarean operation and that if, as the evidence suggested, many of the operations may not have been required, many women were therefore losing their lives unnecessarily. He stated that, in general, the death rate was 5–10 per cent. In the United States the death rate appeared to be lower, but he estimated a death list each year of 900–1,800, with three-quarters of these being unnecessary.

A similar theme was at the heart of a discussion which occurred in 1935 when the *BMJ* had its annual meeting in Melbourne, Australia. Bright Bannister complained that the caesarean operation had degenerated from being an attempt to save lives to an apparently easy way of avoiding difficulties without regard to its perils. There had been an enormous increase in the incidence of the operation often for such slender reasons as failure to progress, advanced age of the mother, breech presentation and unwillingness to undergo the pains of labour. He argued that from the evidence of 1,763 deliveries in large maternity hospitals in England and 1,723 births in Brooklyn occurring between 1921 and 1926, it appeared that the death rate of the mother for caesarean section was 6.6 per cent. For vaginal delivery, it was only 0.45 per cent in England and Wales. He continued to state that in 1932 alone there had been 170 deaths after caesareans. Dr H.A. Ridler of Sydney agreed there were too many caesareans: 'This was the result in modern times of the love of the dramatic, of the desire to earn a big fee easily, and of the love of speed' (Bright Bannister, 1935, p. 685).

However, others argued that in using statistics in this way Bannister was not comparing like with like because women having caesarean were often in a very difficult situation prior to the operation. Professor J.B. Dawson said that in Britain there were not too many caesareans but rather too many done too late. Disasters occurred not after prompt action but after undue delay (Bright Bannister, 1935).

Whilst the *BMJ* and many authorities in the US may have been urging caution in the use of caesarean section, it appears that the rest of the medical profession were determined to fully utilize what they perceived to be the benefits of this method of delivery. The confidence of the medical establishment in caesarean section as a safe operative procedure was highlighted by the fact that the Queen and Princess Margaret entered the world this way in 1926 and 1930 respectively (Holt, 1986).

A new mood of caution

A meeting of the North of England Obstetrical and Gynaecological Society held on the 27th November, 1936 was reported in the *BMJ*. The debate centred on a paper previously presented to the Society by Professor A.M. Claye on the indications for caesarean section. Claye had highlighted the comparatively low mortality from the lower segment operation, even when operations were performed late in labour or after other interventions had been tried. He had further suggested that the operation was safer than craniotomy. Mr W. Gough opened the discussion by criticizing the movement towards the treatment of any obstetric difficulty by section. It is obvious that the medical fraternity had been aware of the risks of widening the number of indications for some time as many of the influential authorities of the time had spoken out urging caution in the employment of the operation. Mr C.M. Marshall, however, stated that the improvements in technique would undoubtedly lead to a wider scope of application and suggested that it would be more productive to explore ways in which the operative technique could be improved. He supported his argument with data from 170 cases of lower segment operations which he had carried out without any maternal deaths. This, of course, was contentious at the time, given the mood of caution sweeping the medical profession regarding the caesarean operation, but the most important aspect of Marshall's contribution to the meeting was that he went on to raise the issue of the use of different types of anaesthesia for abdominal delivery. His contention was that, based on his own experience and results published by Daily from the Chicago Lying-In Hospital, general anaesthesia was much more dangerous to the life of the mother than regional anaesthetic (BMJ, 1936).

The debates of the early twentieth century are important because they represent the first indication that the modern medical profession was beginning to recognize the possible abuse of the operation in terms of it being used in the interests of the practitioner rather than those of the patient. However, such concerns did not result in a reduction in the caesarean section rates. During the Second World War commentators in the United States were still concerned about the levels of caesareans. In 1942 Cotgrove and Norton stated that caesarean section had been frequently used for such reasons as 'primigravidity in the elderly, election by neurotic patients and high social value of the offspring, which can hardly be considered legitimate' (p.201). Delee concurred with these sentiments and commented that the high level of operations was a crucial factor in the continuing high maternal mortality rates (1942).

Thus the debates of the earlier part of the twentieth century demonstrated great concern among some obstetricians about the caesarean rates which were recognized as being above those necessary for the best care of mothers and their babies. Indeed the rates had reached levels where maternal mortality was being increased as a result, rather than decreased.

The role of the Church - part II

Religion continued to have an influence on the practice of childbirth into the twentieth century (as it does today). In fact the Catholic Church was still recommending the performance of caesarean section on the death of the mother right up until the 1930s. In the fifth edition of his book *Moral Problems in Hospital Practice* published in 1935 Finney stated:

> 'The canon directs that, if the mother dies during pregnancy, the fetus should be extracted by those upon whom this duty devolves... the catholic physician is obliged to perform the caesarean operation in all stages of pregnancy beginning with the period when the embryo is distinguishable and has the form of a fetus ... this fourth provision of the canon is based on the fact that the fetus often survives the mother who dies after delivery and therefore nothing should be left undone to extract the fetus without delay, because, under the circumstances there is nearly always the chance to administer baptism and therefore secure eternal life for the fetus.' (p. 46)

In his book, Finney stressed the importance of ensuring that the woman was in fact dead prior to the performance of the operation, as in some cases the woman had been killed by this kind of intervention.

This did not mean that the Catholic Church was not advocating the sacrifice of the mother in order to save the child. In fact, it was quite the reverse. Being totally opposed to the destruction of the infant by procedures such as craniotomy and embryotomy, the Catholic Church recommended that caesareans should be carried out even if it meant the death of the mother. As late as 1935 Papal authority approved the publication in London and St. Louis of the fifth edition of the book *Moral Problems in Hospital Practice* which advocated the sacrifice of the mother rather than saving her life through the destruction of the child. Finney stated:

> 'To preserve ones life is generally speaking duty; but it may be the plainest duty, the highest duty, to sacrifice one's life. War is full of such instances, in which it is not man's duty to live but to die... a parallel case, is the situation of a woman in a difficult labour, when her life and that of her unborn child are in extreme danger. In this situation it is the mother's duty to die rather to consent to the killing of her child.'

He continued:

> 'The first fact in the world is that justice, law and order should be observed no matter what the cost; better that ten thousand mothers should die than one foetus be unjustly killed.' (p. 47)

Finney's book was reviewed in the British medical literature and widely read. He had balanced the life of a fetus with ten thousand women. Others went even further. A.J. Shulte (1917) a professor of Liturgy stated:

'Even if the life of the mother is in danger, a physician has no right to destroy the child's life. I say now and with all seriousness that it is better that one million mothers die than to have one innocent little creature killed.' (p. 52)

Religion continues to have an impact on caesarean section rates in the late twentieth century. In Brazil where the caesarean section rates are the highest in the world at one in three, the Roman Catholic Church's opposition to sterilization has inadvertently increased the number of caesareans. This is because sterilization can be performed at the same time. It has therefore been suggested that many caesarean operations are performed for this reason alone (Faundes and Cecatti, 1993).

New age of 'The Child'

Since 1944 increased emphasis has been placed on perinatal and neonatal outcomes. Before this time interest (outside of the Catholic Church) was concentrated on maternal mortality, whereas fetal and neonatal mortality was seen as a natural part of the childbirth and child-bearing process. The shift in attention reflected changes in attitudes and societal pressures at the time. The end of the Second World War had left most countries with a somewhat depleted population placing greater emphasis on the successful outcome of childbirth. Also, changes taking place in terms of family size with the shift to smaller nuclear units coupled with the introduction of effective birth control in the 1960s had increased emphasis on the outcome of each pregnancy.

The importance placed on the health of the fetus gained more recognition by the mid 1950s and increased its emphasis during the 1960s. With societal pressure for improving the life chances of the fetus and neonate, medical practitioners turned to the caesarean operation in an attempt to address this demand. As emphasis was now being placed on outcome for both mother and fetus/neonate, the medical profession was again forced into the dilemma of having to balance the relative benefits of any interventionist procedure (or lack of it) to each patient.

As caesareans became safer they therefore became more plausible to use. Accompanying this change in emphasis from the older style of interventions in childbirth to the 'new' surgical procedure was a crucial shift in approach, and later attitude, to childbirth, thus there was little overall increase in intervention levels before the 1930s. A decrease in forceps delivery, for example, meant an increase in caesarean section. However, the rise in the caesarean section rates inevitably correlated to increases in the reliance on medical specialists for the management of childbirth. Hence an important implication of the increased use of caesarean section as a mode of delivery was the necessity for hospitalization that accompanied it. By the mid 1950s there was a marked trend towards hospital confinement in the United Kingdom. Hospital deliveries rose from 64 per cent of births in 1955 to 96 per cent in 1974 (O'Brien, 1978). The move towards hospital birth and away from home confinement was based on the assumption that hospitals could offer the safest environment possible for the delivery of infants. An assumption which is still in evidence today, and which continues to be open to question.

Caesareans in the late twentieth century

Recently the increasing use of caesarean section has prompted concern and questions have been raised over the ethicacy of its use. In 1980 the National Institutes of Health (NIH) in the United States held a Health Consensus Development Conference (September 22–24) to address a number of issues relating to caesarean childbirth. The main points of concern were: the increasing rates of caesarean section and reasons for these; the effects of increased use of caesarean section on pregnancy outcomes; the short and long term medical and psychological effects of caesarean delivery on mothers, infants and families; the legal and ethical aspects of decisions to perform caesarean operations and the financial considerations of the rising caesarean rate. After considering the evidence available at that time the task force decided that the increasing rate of caesareans could not be justified in terms of maternal and infant outcomes and was therefore a cause for concern. It went on to stress that the rise could be halted and even reversed while continuing to make improvements in maternal and fetal outcomes. However, it appears that there is still a long way to go to reach an optimum level of caesareans. Writing almost a decade after the NIH report, Myers and Gleicher (1990) stated that part of the NIH report's message had reached some obstetricians but that much of the message had not reached the majority of obstetricians.

In 1993 *Caesarean Birth in Britain* (Francome et al.) was published. This major text raised concern over the rising caesarean rate and effects on women. The number of caesareans performed in this country continues to increase and the rate of increase rises annually. Women are now three times more likely to deliver by caesarean than they were 20 years ago. The important debate over the optimum level of caesareans, absolute indications for the operation and possible effects on women and their children continues today.

CHAPTER EIGHT

Conflict Between Lay and Professional Views on Pregnancy and Labour

This chapter examines different perceptions of childbirth, particularly in relation to the concept of power in maternity services and explores the possibility of gender-related differences in perceptions. Evidence is presented to demonstrate that the conflict has led to a situation where different perceptions of success and satisfaction with childbirth are experienced, often leaving women with no sense of accomplishment or achievement. The theme of conflict is examined through the concepts of power and knowledge, demonstrating that women have been disempowered and deskilled in this situation through the presumed superiority of medical knowledge. It is clear that if women are to be empowered in childbirth, a free exchange of information between pregnant women and professional attendants is required.

There is evidence that medical professionals and women, as consumers of maternity services, have different perceptions about pregnancy and labour. These differences appear to be the result of status differentials between lay people and professionals. They may also be based on gender inequalities. While it is clear that professionals and women as recipients of maternity care services are working towards a common goal, the birth of a healthy baby, the power imbalance has led to a conflict between the two.

Over the years a situation has emerged where opposing perceptions about the meaning of pregnancy and labour are evident and differing levels of knowledge are assumed to exist. Consequently, women and medical professionals had different expectations and experiences of the birth process culminating in differing levels of satisfaction and sense of achievement.

Lay and professional views on childbirth

The process of reproduction may have many connotations. For obstetricians, childbirth can be a small, not terribly significant event in their busy work schedule, that is, it is a 'transient' episode. For women, however, childbirth is a major life event with consequences that stretch far beyond the episode of labour. It is a natural, often inevitable, biological process; an event that has major significance for the whole of their lives, the fulfillment of their expectations and, in some cultures, the fulfillment of society's expectations of them. This conflict in attitude has resulted in women being disempowered in maternity care and the provision of services which may not fully meet their needs.

Women, men and childbirth

Some feminist critiques of the childbirth system have argued that the differing perceptions of childbirth may not be due entirely to differences between lay and professional beliefs but are possibly based upon differences between men and women (Graham and Oakley, 1981). Historically the management of reproduction has been a female concern in most cultures. However, childbirth in industrial societies is characterized by male control. This raises questions about the position of women in general and as child-bearers in particular.

The way in which obstetricians have displaced midwives in the past, and women's loss of control over their own bodies at the time of giving birth has been well documented and it remains a contentious issue.[1] It is not my intention to recount the male take-over of control of pregnancy and childbirth, but rather to highlight the legacy as a result of this power imbalance. Although the majority of deliveries are supervised by midwives in this country, the male-dominated medical frame of reference still threatens the extent to which women in labour can fulfill their hopes and expectations. It has been suggested that the medicalization of childbirth led to the medical profession taking a particular view of women.

> 'The conversion of female controlled community management to male controlled medical management alone would suggest that the propagation of particular paradigms of women as maternity cases has been central to the whole development of medically dominated maternity care.' (Oakley, 1980, p. 11)

Gender theory has been successfully employed in the analysis of lay and professional views on childbirth and can demonstrate how cognitive differences between men and women contribute to high levels of unnecessary intervention in labour including caesarean section. For example the obstetric discourse is based upon 'masculine' or 'scientific' models, whereby emotional detachment and objectivity are believed to ensure accurate observation and/or diagnosis. However, the female frame of reference emphasizes the maintenance of relationships and personal connection with knowledge rather than detachment from it. Thus women may distrust the scientific, detached approach and perceive obstetricians to be uncaring. These opposing perspectives conflict in the labour ward and can lead to anxiety for women which may affect the birth process leading to more intervention (LoCicero, 1993).[2]

---

1. See Ehrenrich, B., English, D. (1979). *For Her Own Good, 150 Years of the Experts' Advice to Women.* London: Pluto Press. This gives a detailed account of male professionals' take-over of skills and knowledge traditionally the domain of women.
2. For a full account of how childbirth intervention (and caesarean section) rates can be analyzed in terms of gender theory, see LoCicero, A.K. (1993). 'Explaining excessive rates of cesareans and other childbirth interventions: contributions from contemporary theories of gender and psychosocial development'. *Social Science and Medicine*, 37(10), pp. 1261–1269.

It could be argued that as a percentage of doctors are also women, any difference between the ideas and expectations of obstetricians and pregnant women cannot be analyzed in terms of gender. It is, however, useful to bear in mind that women doctors are in a patriarchal profession. They have been trained with men's knowledge about women and women's bodies, and it is inevitable that they will have internalized at least some male medical attitudes and perceptions.

Midwives have been in a different position altogether. While predominantly a female profession, midwifery remains part of the medical establishment. Some midwives experience regret when obstetricians take over the birth process and sympathize with women over their sense of loss when technology is used to achieve delivery (Inch, 1986), but others have accepted the medical model of pregnancy and childbirth, seeing a successful outcome as a healthy baby, regardless of the means by which it was achieved.

> 'If at the end of the day (or night) a healthy baby is born into the world, is it such an earth-shaking tragedy that a caesarean section was used to bring this about?' (Holt, 1986, p. 60)

Some women (and men) are breaking free from this dominant male interpretation of knowledge and are spearheading the way forward to a woman-centred approach to obstetric care. But at what individual cost are such changes being made? One has only to look at the case of Wendy Savage in 1985 to appreciate the strength of opposition to any challenge to technological management and medical models of care in obstetrics.[3]

Power in childbirth

Power is an important element in the differing experiences and expectations of the medical profession and women as receivers of maternity care. There is an unequal relationship between the two, in which doctors still generally hold the power. Women are expected to be passive in the labour theatre, with insufficient information to make choices about their care. This system leads to feelings of frustration, powerlessness and alienation from the conduct of childbirth.

Historically, the medical definition of care demanded that patients be compliant and obedient. A study from the US demonstrated how women questioning the decisions of doctors were met with hostility:

> 'I never saw the baby when it came out. I kept asking to see the baby while I was fighting to keep my eyes open. The doctor said to me, "I have never seen someone complain so much at such a happy occasion". I wasn't complaining; I was asking to see my baby.' (Perez, 1989, p. 137)

---

3. Wendy Savage, Consultant Obstetrician at the London Hospital, was suspended from work in 1985 following the death of a neonate for not performing a caesarean section in a situation where her colleagues would have (see Savage, W. (1986). *A Savage Enquiry*. London: Virago Press).

On the other hand, if women request interventionist techniques, this is accepted as 'legitimate patient behaviour'. By requesting intervention the woman has been viewed as displaying two important aspect of patient behaviour: first, accepting the notion that medical control and intervention equals good (safe) childbirth, and secondly, accepting the doctor's superior knowledge and expertise (Graham and Oakley, 1981). The technological management of childbirth also enables doctors to exert power over other professional groups within the hospital hierarchy. When the decision is made to use technology to deliver a child, control is taken out of the hands of everyone except the obstetricians. Midwives may therefore experience a sense of loss and regret at having to relinquish control and assume an assisting role in the birth process (Inch, 1986).

The conflict between lay and professional views on pregnancy and labour has resulted in differing experiences of delivery in terms of satisfaction and sense of achievement.

Success in childbirth

Success may be perceived differently by obstetricians and women in childbirth. Obstetricians tend to view 'success' in terms of perinatal and maternal mortality rates. They may not therefore understand the sense of disappointment that some women experience following delivery, even when the outcome is a healthy baby.

For women 'success' in terms of pregnancy and childbirth is a more complex issue. Of course, the birth of a healthy baby is of paramount importance in almost all cases, but for many women 'success' is also measured in terms of a personally satisfying experience and sense of achievement. The physical and emotional exhaustion of a possibly long labour that culminates in technological intervention and even surgery cannot be underestimated. It is suggested that such events may result in a process of grieving which can go on for months and even years (Laufer et al., 1987).

This is not to deny the experiences of many women who find childbirth a rewarding and fulfilling event, but rather to point to the dissatisfaction of some women with the medical model of pregnant women and interventionist approaches to childbirth. It is possible that as rates of intervention increase, less and less women will have rewarding experiences of childbirth. It would be unrealistic to suggest that labour is an ideal process during which women need no help or support. Interventions clearly do save lives. However, the problem is what many view as the over-use of interventionist techniques which may only be required in selected cases. Thus the current pattern of medical intervention in childbirth is not necessarily in the best interest of women and their babies.

Satisfaction with childbirth

Increasingly intervention in childbirth, together with other medical fashions such as routine episiotomy and fetal monitoring, led to women being disempowered during maternity care and becoming reliant on the expertise of the professionals. Women are still enveloped by the medical model of childbirth which may be at odds with their own wishes concerning labour and delivery. Critics of the system have suggested that it has inculcated in women the expectation of relinquishing their will, their power and potentially their rights to an uncaring, mechanistic, process-orientated system where they will accept without question interventionist techniques (Graham and Oakley, 1981).

There is a wealth of evidence relating to women who are dissatisfied with their experiences of childbirth. Correlations were found between technological intervention in childbirth and feelings of depression among women after giving birth (Oakley, 1980). Thus technology has deprived women of a fulfilling start to motherhood, leaving them dissatisfied, disappointed, with no sense of achievement.

Some argue that if there is any satisfaction to be gained from the interventionist approach to labour, it is doctors who experience it, in the form of job satisfaction from the use of high technology. In other words, professionals gain satisfaction from the exercise of their skills and knowledge, at the expense of women's satisfaction with the childbirth experience.

Knowledge about childbirth

The medicalization of women's bodies established childbirth as a specialist field where only doctors have appropriate knowledge. The notion that the medical profession possess superior knowledge in matters relating to childbirth has been consistently opposed by commentators suggesting that childbearing is something that women do have knowledge about, as they are, after all, the ones with the physiological equipment for reproduction.

It has been argued that women have 'intuitive knowledge (about pregnancy and childbirth) built up from bodily experiences' (Graham and Oakley, 1981, p. 55). There is evidence to support this view. It appears that when women do refuse interventions, because of their knowledge about pregnancy, childbirth and their own bodies, they are likely to deliver a perfectly healthy baby normally (Woodcraft, 1988). But there are two factors at work here which act against women accepting or expressing their own knowledge. First, when women do display knowledge, intuitive or experiential, about their bodies, this can be ignored by the medical attendants at the birth as the results of a study from the US have shown:

> 'When they sat me up for the epidural, I really felt like pushing and kept saying, "Wait, wait a minute. I need to push". They ignored me and gave me the epidural.'

This woman was then given a caesarean. She commented:

> 'As soon as they finished stitching me up I knew I wouldn't do this again. For some reason, even then, I knew I could have given birth normally.' (Perez, 1989, p. 138)

Secondly, I would argue that the medicalization process has stripped women of their knowledge, expertise and their confidence in dealing with pregnancy and childbirth. Women have, in a sense, relinquished the will to take care of themselves to the higher authority of the medical profession, a form of cultural iatrogenesis. A respondent in Perez's study commented: 'I didn't ask any questions. I just trusted everyone. I felt they must know what they were doing' (1989, p. 131).

Women's acceptance of medical domination of knowledge in childbirth is dramatically illustrated by one of the participants in Sargent and Stark's study (in the United States) of women's reactions to caesarean birth. The woman who had delivered two previous babies vaginally arrived at the hospital informing the staff that she was in labour but was told that she was not. Not only did the woman know from her previous experiences that she was in labour, she was also aware that this particular labour was not normal. The staff disagreed and told her not to worry. Eventually the woman was given a caesarean. When interviewed by the researchers about the events leading to the surgical delivery the woman complained that the doctors and nurses treated her as if she did not know anything about her own body. But, when asked if she felt that the medical staff should have taken her opinions more seriously she said 'no', because after all, 'the doctor is the specialist' (1987, p. 1272).

This demonstrates that when women do have knowledge about pregnancy and childbirth, whether this be intuitive or experiential, when they are confident and articulate in asserting their knowledge about their own bodies, they often bow to the superior knowledge of the medical authorities who are seen to be the experts in matters relating to the human body.

This evidence clearly shows an acceptance of the medicalization of birth and possible expectation of technological intervention at delivery. It further demonstrates the fact that the doctors have successfully inculcated the notion that they are the ones with the expertise in childbirth in their own minds and the minds of those in whose interest they should be working – the women. This is further highlighted by the fact that when women do not receive all the information they require during childbirth, they tend, on the whole, to be very satisfied with the care and information they have received. This implies that when information is not given to women it is perceived by those women to be not relevant or unnecessary, after all, 'doctor knows best'. The expression of satisfaction among women after failure to obtain the information required highlights the subtlety of the exercise of power implicit in the doctor-patient relationship (Shapiro et al., 1983).

The medical profession's overwhelming sense of ownership of knowledge about pregnancy and childbirth has been dramatically highlighted in the United States with doctors requesting, and often receiving, the backing of the courts to perform caesarean sections on women who have refused to grant consent for the operation (Brahams, 1988; Morgan, 1992).

This sort of court order made 'on behalf of the fetus' is not unusual in the States and the possibility of such orders being made in Britain is not as remote as we might expect. Towards the end of 1987 barristers were briefed by a local authority to advise on ways of obtaining an order requiring a woman to go to hospital and, if necessary, undergo a caesarean section (Woodcraft, 1988). On 13 October 1992 a woman was forced to undergo a caesarean section against her wishes. She had objected on religious grounds and her partner agreed to and supported her decision. However, the obstetrician responsible for this case had convinced the High Court that the baby would die if the caesarean was not performed. This is the first case in modern times where the rights of the unborn child have taken precedence over the rights of the mother to determine her treatment (Crafter, 1994). A news item appeared in the press on 16 September 1996 relating to two cases which arose on the same day in June. A judge of the High Court's family court decided that doctors could perform caesarean sections on two women in labour who had refused the operation. His reasoning being that the women were incapable of making the decision while in stressful and painful labour. Such evidence indicates not only the unequivocal sense of ownership of knowledge and expertise among the medical profession regarding childbirth, to the extent that women's rights of consent are overruled in favour of doctors' decisions, but also highlights the pervasiveness of such an ideology and its exercise in other patriarchal institutions. Women's knowledge or preferences were not considered here. The positions of the women in this case were not heard in court.

The trend continues despite the paucity of evidence to justify such action in terms of maternal, perinatal or neonatal outcomes. A national survey in the United States in 1987 found 15 cases of attempts to legally enforce caesarean sections. Thirteen of the 15 requests were granted by the courts. Only two of the babies delivered by these operations were actually found to be ill after delivery. Given the higher mortality and morbidity rates associated with abdominal birth it could be argued that court-ordered interventions adversely affect maternal and infant health and demonstrate that the presumed authority of the medical profession is not necessarily in the interests of women and their babies.

Clearly the majority of women do not have the benefit of a medical education and, as such, cannot make decisions based on medical criteria alone. However, women do have varying degrees of intuitive knowledge about their bodies and many have experiential knowledge about pregnancy and labour. If women are to gain their rightful position in the decision-making process, a sharing of knowledge and information is required. This can only be achieved if medical professionals impart knowledge to their patients in order for them to make informed decisions.

The right to information

One very important process by which the power imbalance between doctors and women as lay recipients of care is maintained is through the amount and quality of information which is exchanged. The sharing of information can be seen as equivalent to sharing power, while withholding information means that the doctor maintains complete control.

For women to achieve a sense of participation in childbirth they need to be informed of what is happening to them during the delivery. Appropriate information during childbirth is equated with more positive experiences overall for women giving birth. Evidence from the US suggests that women's satisfaction with their experience of labour and delivery is frequently related to whether or not they feel that they have received enough information (Shapiro et al., 1983; Fawcett and Burritt, 1985). However, many women were unhappy with the amount of information they received (Shapiro, 1983). Lack of information during delivery affects women's perceptions of the birth process.

A UK study of maternal satisfaction found that over three quarters (77 per cent) of the women who said that they had received insufficient information were dissatisfied with the management of their labour and delivery (Martin, 1990).

The evidence available points to the fact that the conflict between lay and professional perceptions leads to a breakdown of communication. It appears that obstetricians, in particular, are unaware of the amount and nature of information that should be exchanged. Shapiro et al. found that obstetricians in the US underestimated the amount of information required by women and, not surprisingly therefore, the majority of women did not receive all the information they wanted (Shapiro et al., 1983).

Evidence from the States has further highlighted a major concern. It has been suggested that the ethos of professionals as 'experts' gives them the right to carry out procedures which are often quite intrusive without explanation and that women asking questions about treatment and/or their condition are seen as 'difficult' rather than simply wanting to know what is happening (Perez, 1989). Thus there appears to be an attitude among medical professionals that women either do not need to know all the details about their condition or that they will not understand the medical implications even if they are given the information.

Giving the wrong information

It appears that when attempts are made to inform women about their condition and treatment the correct message does not always get across and women are left at best, partially informed and, at worst, misinformed. Evidence suggests that when women are given information during delivery they may not be given the correct information and there may not be agreement between medical staff over the facts of the case so that women are inappropriately informed (Perez, 1989). Further, it has been found that women who have caesarean births often do not know why the caesareans were performed, give the wrong explanation when compared to their medical notes or are only partially correct in their explanations (Hillan, 1992). Similarly, discrepancies have been found between the treatment that women receive and the treatment that is recorded in their medical notes (Perez, 1989).

Withholding information

A common way that women are denied knowledge about their condition and treatment is by the withholding of information. Evidence from the States suggests that women were given medication against their wishes and that treatment was administered without allowing women choice (Perez, 1989). Obviously if women are to make decisions regarding their treatment in hospital it is imperative that they receive appropriate and accurate information. The withholding of information indicates a misuse of power by the professionals. Women can not have a say in what happens to them if they do not know the details of their condition. Withholding information is therefore a very effective way for the power imbalance to be maintained.

It is clear that the conflict between lay and professional views on labour and delivery stem from assumptions about the possession of knowledge in childbirth which are maintained by the control of information. Lack of information-sharing within obstetric care is not the result of willful neglect but rather a combination of factors including confusion over whose responsibility it is to inform women in this situation.

Changing childbirth: has the conflict been resolved?

The report 'Changing Childbirth' (DOH, 1993) provided the blueprint for a change in midwifery and obstetric practice to a more woman-centred approach and could lead to a resolution of the conflict between lay and professional views and experience of childbirth.

The main recommendations of the report were that women should be provided with adequate information to enable decision-making regarding care and that continuity of care is essential for the communication between professionals and their patients.

Informed consent

The notion of consent to medical intervention in childbirth becomes a nonsense if women are not adequately informed. For example, when women are asked to consent to an emergency caesarean operation, they may do so without really understanding what the procedures entail. In such cases it is questionable whether the consent given by the woman represents a free choice. Women can have no time to reflect in such cases. They may be manipulated by the professional's concentration on delivery as a potential disaster, feel forced into the hospital's 'surgical agenda', or feel pressurized into conforming to the expectations of the patient role in what could be, after all, an emergency situation. It is a nonsense therefore to expect women to be prepared for such circumstances.

Thus it is the responsibility of health care professionals to impart to women and their partners, information that is accurate and offered at a level that is accessible to the individuals concerned. This is to empower them to participate in the decision-making process and to enable them to feel as though they have taken a meaningful role in the birth of their children.

Whose role is it to inform women?

Evidence from Britain (Martin, 1990; DOH, 1993) and the States (Fawcett and Burritt, 1985; Shapiro et al., 1983) has shown that many women are dissatisfied with the amount of information that they receive during childbirth and that this affects their perceptions and sense of participation in the birth process.

One possible explanation for women being ill-informed about their treatment is that there is confusion among hospital staff in terms of who has responsibility for informing women of all that is happening. What this means is that women are told nothing or very little, as all staff believe that someone else has already taken responsibility for informing them. Hillan found that some women in her study said that they were never told directly why their caesareans were necessary but picked up snippets of information from overheard conversations between the medical staff (1992).

One of the reasons why women may be ill-informed during delivery is that there is not always agreement between different professional groups as to the details of the case (Perez, 1989). It is not surprising, therefore, that women are either not given enough information or are inappropriately informed about their condition when differences exist between perceptions of the case by different professionals.

Another explanation is that, while giving information to women, the hospital staff are fulfilling their professional obligations, but it does not guarantee that the patient understands the exact nature of the treatment and the implications of it.

Information given by medical practitioners may not always be adequate, perhaps because of insufficient time and because medical terminology can be poorly understood by patients. Or it may be that at the time the decision to perform the caesarean was made the women may not have been in a position to fully understand (Hillan, 1992). Obstetrician Wendy Savage has suggested that as a woman in hospital tends to meet several different professionals who she does not know who may explain things differently from those who know her and at the wrong level, this is likely to increase anxiety for the patient and could lead to misunderstandings (1986).

'Changing Childbirth' places midwives at the centre of the information-providing process. Such a suggestion is not new. Vocal midwives have been arguing for a more active role for many years. Similarly, almost 20 years ago it was suggested that midwives were in a position to ensure that women have a more dominant and less subservient role in the delivery process. They can facilitate communication between women and their doctors and ensure that the women's needs are not ignored or suppressed (Cartwright, 1979). The suggestion is that whereas decisions about whether to perform the caesarean, which anaesthetic to use and whether the partner should be allowed into the operating theatre, are made by the physician, information given to women about caesarean birth can be controlled by nurses and therefore they need to take a more active role in ensuring that women are fully informed (Fawcett, 1990). This may be possible when medical staff have time but in an emergency situation it could be very different. Sally Inch suggests that although speed is essential, the midwife knows that the faster things happen the more alarming it will be for the woman and her partner. There is therefore a potential for explanations about the preparation and procedure of surgery to be hurried and thus unlikely to be taken in by the woman and/or her partner (1986). However, it appears that in the past, even when the nursing staff did take an active role in giving information to caesarean patients this was not always in the interest of the women concerned. Hillan found lack of support and conflicting advice from midwives, especially in postnatal wards (1992).

The 'Changing Childbirth' document has now had time to make an impact but many believe that change has yet to take place. Some scepticism has been voiced from within the midwifery profession over midwives' competence, ability and willingness to take on board the recommendations (Cardale, 1994). It may be that the medical model has dominated for too long and has inculcated in the minds of lay people and maternity professionals the view of childbirth as pathological (Clarke, 1994). A change in attitude among midwives is therefore required if change in practice is to be possible (Browne, 1994; Cardale, 1994; Clarke, 1994; Flint, 1994) and this may necessitate a degree of re-training that, in many instances, is yet to be provided (Davis, 1994).

Is continuity of care a possibility?

It was encouraging to see that 'Changing Childbirth' recommended continuity of maternity care carried out primarily by midwives. This represented a long-awaited recognition among an 'expert maternity group' of the importance of continuity of care. Continuity of care before, during and after caesarean delivery is much less common than with vaginal delivery (Inch, 1986). This may be one reason why women having caesareans tend to report less satisfaction with the birth process than those delivering vaginally. Where women do receive continuity of care they are more likely to rate their antenatal care as 'good' or 'very good' (Martin, 1990).

Communication and sharing of information can be impeded by the fact that women have seen different practitioners each time they attend the hospital for antenatal check-ups. This is a problem for the women in particular because they were not able to develop relationships with their physicians. The majority of women prefer continuity of care during pregnancy, that is, they wish to be able to see the same doctor or midwife throughout. Yet, in the past, very few have received it (Martin, 1990). However, to provide continuity of care midwives will need to change not simply their attitudes but also their working practices (Flint, 1994).

The future?

Obstetricians are educated to identify and treat complications in labour. They are also trained in the use of technology to aid the birth process. Obviously many lives are saved because of these skills. However, it is surely time that obstetricians are allowed to concentrate on the small minority of women who require their skills and expertise while the majority of women in labour are supervised by the custodians of normality in childbirth, the midwives.

'Changing Childbirth' recognized this fact and made recommendations placing midwives at the centre of maternity care. However, it may be a case of 'too little, too late'. Obstetric domination of maternity care over the past three decades could mean that midwives have been deskilled (Clarke, 1994) and that a period of re-training may be essential before the recommendation can be fully implemented (Davis, 1994).

It is clear that the conflict between lay and professional views on labour and delivery has led to very different perceptions of childbirth and experiences of success and satisfaction. The position is exacerbated by status (power) differentials and by an assumed superiority of medical knowledge. There is evidence that a crucial determinant of satisfaction with maternity care, at all stages, is the quality of the communication between women and the professional staff.

Over ten years ago the WHO stated:

> 'The training of health professionals should include communication techniques in order to promote sensitive exchange of information between members of the health team and the pregnant woman and her family.' (1985, p. 436)

Yet the evidence available suggests that the conflicting perceptions between obstetricians and women in childbirth continue to hinder communication, thus leading to a less satisfactory experience for women. Therefore, not only does the medical profession need to be encouraged to impart information to women to empower them to participate in decision-making, but also health practitioners need to ensure that the information given to women is accurate and imparted at a level that is accessible to the individuals concerned. Only then will a 'successful' and 'satisfying' outcome be reached by women as well as by the medical practitioners and thereby some resolution to the conflict between lay and professional views on pregnancy and labour be achieved.

CHAPTER NINE

Caesarean Birth Today

Caesarean section rates

Rates of caesarean section have been rising in all countries where data is available (apart from the United States which has experienced a decline in recent years). In Britain the caesarean rate rose from 2.7 per cent of all births in 1958 to 15.3 per cent in 1993 (Savage and Francome, 1993; Francome, 1994).

Regional variations

Overall rates for caesarean section mask significant regional variations. A study in Great Britain found that the caesarean rates in England ranged from 10.1 per cent in the South Western region to 12.9 per cent in South East Thames. All the Thames regions had rates of 12.2 per cent or above whereas Trent, North Western and Northern had rates below 11.4 per cent. Scotland had a rate of 14.2 per cent and for Wales it was 13.5 per cent. However, most of the Welsh Health Authorities had rates below 13 per cent, yet two had rates of 14 per cent and one had an unprecedented 17.5 per cent caesarean section rate (Savage and Francome, 1993).

Caesarean section rates also vary between hospitals from 9.4 per cent in a Liverpool hospital to 22.7 per cent in one London hospital (Francome, 1994). On the whole, teaching hospitals appear to have much higher caesarean section rates than non-teaching hospitals. The most frequently cited reason for the difference is that teaching hospitals are more likely to treat 'high risk' women who have been referred to them. However, this does not appear to be the case as there are marked differences in caesarean rates between teaching hospitals and, more specifically, between those hospitals in London and those in other areas, whereas the range of complications are likely to be the same. Furthermore, in Scotland there is little difference between caesarean rates for teaching hospitals and non-teaching hospitals, despite the increased referral rate of higher risk patients to the teaching hospitals (Savage and Francome, 1993).

Such regional and hospital variations cannot be accounted for in terms of differences in the population of women served by these regions or hospitals, but rather to differences in obstetrical practice and policy. This point is further highlighted by the fact that the Dumfries and Galloway area had a caesarean section rate of 15.8 per cent in 1985, yet during 1986, while cases were being scrutinized and interest in the rising incidence of caesarean section was high, the rate dropped to 11.6 per cent (Urquhart et al., 1987), suggesting that factors other than medical necessity were affecting the number of caesareans being performed.

Socio-economic factors

Where population differences in caesarean section rates are evident (as in the United States), they are closely related to social class and appear to follow an inverse care law, that is, the lower the social class, the higher the medical risk and the lower the medical attention and treatment available (Chalmers and Richards, 1977; Hurst and Summey, 1984). Therefore it is the wealthier women who are receiving more caesarean sections than their counterparts in the lower socio-economic groupings. In the United States this class differential is related to the difference between private and public health care with the caesarean section rates for private hospitals being substantially higher than those of public hospitals. In 1986 the caesarean section rate in the United States was 24.4 per cent. Women with private insurance had the highest caesarean section rate at 29.1 per cent (Stafford, 1990; Taffel et al., 1992).

In Brazil, nearly 32 per cent of all babies are delivered by caesarean section (Taffel et al., 1992). A 1984 study demonstrated the marked differences in caesarean section rates for women in the different socio-economic groups. The rate was 7.5 per cent among the poor, uninsured women; 9.5 per cent among publicly insured; and 49.6 per cent among the wealthier private patients (Janowitz et al., 1984). More recently in the private clinics in urban areas the caesarean section rate was almost 90 per cent (Macnair, 1992).

It appears that England and Wales are following the American example. Almost twenty years ago Ann Cartwright demonstrated that the induction rate of women in the private sector was twice the national average (1979) and it was suggested that a similar finding would emerge from analysis of the caesarean section rates (Richards, 1979). Evidence is now available to support this view. In 1980 women having babies in National Health Service (NHS) hospitals were found to have a caesarean rate of nine per cent whilst women in pay-beds (private) within the NHS hospitals had a rate of 19.6 per cent (Macfarlane and Mugford, 1986). Similar trends are evident in the rest of Europe. In the Lazio region of Italy a strong relationship was found between mode of hospital payment and the caesarean section rate. Women in the private hospitals had the highest rates at 34.7 per cent whilst the National Health Service public hospitals had a rate of 21.3 per cent (Bertollini et al., 1992). A study in Spain also found caesarean rates to be significantly higher in private hospitals (Santamera and Gutierrez, 1994).

Ownership of private insurance also seems to affect whether women will have a vaginal birth after caesarean (VBAC) as this occurs more than twice as frequently in women not covered by private insurance (Stafford, 1990). The implication here is that, as surgical birth is more lucrative, caesareans are being performed rather than allowing women a trial of labour for subsequent pregnancies.

What this points to, once again, is that caesarean section rates are not dependent upon medical necessity but are, in this case, the result of socio-economic factors.

Caesarean rates and perinatal/neonatal outcomes

While the caesarean section rates have risen in most countries for which data is available, perinatal outcomes have improved significantly. This has led to the suggestion that there is a direct causal relationship between high caesarean rates and lower perinatal mortality rates. However, the reduction in perinatal and neonatal mortality rates can be explained in other ways, the most likely explanation being better overall living conditions and levels of health in those populations experiencing better perinatal outcomes.

The high caesarean section rate cannot be justified in terms of reductions in perinatal and neonatal mortality. While caesarean section rates increased in the United States for many years, there was no evidence to suggest that this had any effect on the infant mortality rate (Shearer, 1993). Despite technological advances in childbirth intervention in the United States, infant mortality rates have remained behind those of other industrialized countries (Romalis, 1985).

Holland in the early 1980s had only a fifth of the United States' caesarean rate but a much lower infant death rate (Francome, 1990). In Dublin, over a 15 year period, perinatal mortality rates improved parallel to those in the United States, although the incidence of caesarean section remained substantially unchanged in Dublin and quadrupled in North America. Infant deaths dropped from 42 per 1000 live births to 17 per 1000 live births, while the caesarean section rate remained constant at between 4 and 5 per cent (O'Driscoll and Foley, 1983). Similarly in New York City between 1967–8 and 1976–7 neonatal mortality decreased markedly, particularly in the section of infants weighing between 1000–2500 grams. The decrease in the neonatal mortality rate for this group of infants, however, was common to both primary caesarean and vaginal births. The decreases could be due to other factors such as improvements in neonatal intensive care. For births above 2500 grams the decrease in neonatal mortality was slight:

> 'No decrease was found in neonatal mortality among all primary cesarean births when allowing for shifts that may have occurred from forceps to cesarean delivery.' (NIH, 1981, p. 175)

Similarly another North American study of caesarean section rates covering a 20 year period (1968–87) found that the five-fold annual increase in the section rate had contributed little, if anything, to reductions in fetal and neonatal mortality during that time (Sepkowitz, 1992). Thus there is no reason to suggest that an increase in the caesarean rate is a causal factor in the decrease in perinatal or neonatal mortality.

Further, it appears that perinatal and neonatal outcomes can be improved whilst reducing rates of caesarean section. The University Medical Center of Jacksonville (Florida) accomplished a reduction in its caesarean section rates whilst improving perinatal and neonatal outcomes over a four-year period of study (Sanchez-Ramos et al., 1990). Similarly, the Hintom Medical Clinic, Alta, Canada, reduced its caesarean section rate from 23 per cent in 1985 to 13 per cent in 1989 without compromising perinatal mortality figures (Inglesias et al., 1992). In areas where perinatal mortality is particularly high, increased use of caesarean section does not appear to have affected perinatal deaths (Mukherjee et al., 1993). What the evidence does suggest is that beyond a caesarean rate of 6 per cent no improvements in perinatal or neonatal outcomes are achieved (Francome and Huntingford, 1980).

It therefore appears that high caesarean rates do not lead to lower rates of infant death and it has been suggested that perinatal outcomes may even be compromised by surgical delivery (Porreco, 1985; Lomas and Enkin, 1989; Rydhström et al., 1990). One Vienna Clinic adopted a non-interventionist policy regarding the treatment of women in labour which resulted in a caesarean section rate ten times lower than the rest of Vienna where technical aids were widely used in all hospitals. Researchers found that the perinatal mortality rates for the clinic were not higher, and the maternal and postneonatal mortality rates were significantly lower than the corresponding rates for Vienna (Rockenschaub, 1990). Evidence therefore refutes claims that childbirth is made safer by the application of high technology and demonstrates that a less interventionist approach can lead to better perinatal mortality rates. What the evidence does suggest is that the rising caesarean section rate is linked to factors which do not relate to the population of women concerned or the desire to keep perinatal and neonatal mortality rates at the lowest possible level.

International comparison of caesarean section rates

Increase in caesarean section rates is an international phenomena, although there are marked differences in the rates between countries (see Table 9.1). Brazil has the highest rate of caesareans in the world where nearly one in three (32 per cent) of births are abdominal. Puerto Rico has the next highest rate of caesareans where three in ten (29 per cent) births are by caesarean. The United States has the third highest level with nearly one birth in four being an operative delivery (Taffel et al., 1992). This, despite the World Health Organization (WHO) statement in 1985:

> 'Countries with some of the lowest perinatal mortality rates in the world have caesarean section rates of less than 10 per cent. There is no justification for any region to have a rate higher than 10–15 per cent.' (p. 437)

Although the rate of caesarean is highest in the Americas, one thing is clear – rising caesarean section rates are an international phenomena (see Figure 9.1).

Some of the lowest rates of caesarean section have been identified in European countries, Holland being the lowest with 7.9 per cent in 1991 (Treffers and Pel, 1993), the rate for Czechoslovakia was 8.1 per cent in 1988, although Jamaica had a caesarean rate of 5.4 per cent in the late 1980s (Webster et al., 1992). The best estimates for Australia indicate that the percentage of deliveries by caesarean rose from 4.2 per cent in 1970 to 16.9 per cent in 1986 (Renwick, 1991) (These figures are estimates as there are no uniform sources of data providing national figures for caesarean rates in Australia.) The primary caesarean section rate in Tasmania rose from 4.3 per cent in 1975 to 6.6 per cent in 1982 (Murray-Arthur and Correy, 1984). Italy experienced an increase in caesarean section rates from 11.2 per cent in 1980 to 17.5 per cent in 1987 (Savage and Francome, 1993) and Spain an increase from 9.9 per cent to 20.0 per cent from 1984 to

1988 (Santamera and Gutierrez, 1994). In Canada the caesarean rate rose from 5.7 per cent in 1970 to 19.9 per cent in 1988 (Lomas and Enkin, 1989; Nair, 1991). In Scotland the caesarean section rate rose steadily from 4.7 per cent in 1970 to 12.8 per cent in 1982 and 14.0 per cent in 1989 (McIlwaine et al., 1985; Francome et al., 1993).

Country	1970	1975	1980	1981	1982	1983	1985	1986	1987	1988	1989	1990
Australia	4.2	8.2	13.2					16.9				
Austria					7.0	7.5						
Belgium					8.0	8.1			9.8			
Canada	5.7	9.6	16.1							19.9		
Czech.	2.3	2.8	4.4		5.2	6.0				8.1		
Denmark	5.7	7.5	10.7		11.7	12.8						
England	4.9				8.2		10.5				12.0	
Fiji			5.2		5.3							
Finland	6.0	8.2								14.4		
France	6.0			10.9								
Greece											16.7	
Holland	2.1	2.7	4.7		5.3		6.3		6.8	7.2		
Hungary	6.2	6.5			9.2					10.2		
Ireland					6.2							
Israel					10.0					10.2		
Italy		11.2				14.5			17.5			
Japan				8.0								
NZ	3.9				9.8							
Norway	2.2	4.1	7.2		9.0	9.4						
Portugal							11.1		14.1	15.5	16.5	
Scotland	4.7	8.1	11.7		12.8				12.8	13.8	14.0	
Singapore			14.7									
Spain						9.9		11.7	12.5	20.0		
Sweden		7.8	12.0									
Tasmania		4.3			6.6							
USA	5.5	10.4	16.5		18.5	20.3	22.7		24.4	24.7	23.8	23.5
Wales					10.6				12.3	12.4	13.4	

(Sources: Australia: Renwick, 1991; Canada: Lomas and Enkin, 1989, Nair, 1991; Italy: Savage and Francome, 1993; Scotland: McIlwaine et al., 1985, Francome et al., 1993; Spain: Santamera and Gutierrez, 1994; Tasmania: Murray-Arthur and Correy, 1984; All others: Francome et al., 1993).

Table 9.1: Some international rates of caesarean section, 1979 to 1990

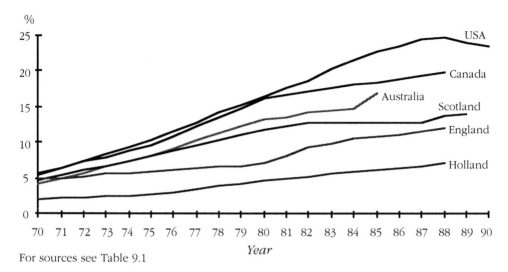

For sources see Table 9.1

Fig. 9.1: Some international rates of caesarean section, 1970 to 1990

Despite having the highest caesarean section rate with nearly 32 per cent of all babies being born by caesarean section, the Brazilian rate is also expected to rise. One estimation put it at 60 per cent by the year 2000 (Macnair, 1992). Although this seems excessive and rates are unlikely to rise that high, such speculations may serve as a warning about what might happen if caesarean rates are permitted to increase unchecked.

However, national figures tend to conceal marked differences relating to areas and hospitals. For example, whilst the caesarean rate for Italy in 1987 was 17.5 per cent, the Lazio region had a rate of 24.3 per cent (Bertollini et al., 1992). Similarly whilst the overall rate for Wales was 13.5 per cent in 1992, the rate for one region was 17.5 per cent (Savage and Francome, 1993). Although some population differences do exist, these cannot account for the overall difference in caesarean rates.

It appears that differences in rates reflect differences in obstetric practice rather than differences in the populations of women served. The dramatic difference between caesarean delivery rates has been ascribed in particular to differences in the management of dystocia and of women who have had previous caesarean deliveries. For example, in 1981 the rate of VBAC was only five per cent in the United States but 43 per cent in Norway (Notzon et al., 1987). Similarly when the rates of caesarean section for all births (and not only births in hospitals) are taken into consideration, the Netherlands emerges as having the lowest rate with only five per cent of births by caesarean. What is interesting about these data is that unlike other developed countries where less than two per cent of deliveries are home births, in the Netherlands a third of all births take place at home (Notzon et al., 1987). Similarly in Holland, the yearly two per cent decline in home births in favour of hospitalization has been directly linked to greater reliance on obstetricians and inevitably, increased rates of intervention including caesarean section (Guillemin, 1981). What this demonstrates is that international caesarean rates are dependent on factors such as hospitalization, medical tradition and obstetricians' preference rather than strict medical necessity.

Caesarean section in the developing world

Although data on caesarean section rates in developing countries is less rigourously collected than in other areas, some trends are identifiable. For those countries where data are available it appears that the caesarean rates are comparable to, or even higher than those reported in developed countries (Notzon et al., 1987). However, there are other factors to consider here. In some cultures women who cannot deliver vaginally are stigmatized. For example, in rural Eastern Nigeria women fear caesarean section as they might be considered abnormal for not being able to deliver vaginally. Caesarean section is also threatening to them because they fear blood transfusion or involuntary sterilization (practiced in some hospitals after repeat caesareans). To those women a caesarean section may mean more than the delivery of a healthy baby or the saving of their lives. The abdominal scar will act as a constant reminder of their incapacity to deliver vaginally. Women may be considered 'mutilated' by those who represent western customs and ignore traditional concepts (Engelkes and van Roosmalen, 1992). As recently as 1993 a paper in the *Journal of the Pakistan Medical Association* recommended craniotomy as opposed to caesarean section for 'selected cases', the authors' rationale being that 'though unpleasant to perform, is of great relief to the patient and her family' (Tariq and Korejo, 1993). Therefore, although some similarity in increasing caesarean section rates can be observed, the reasoning and the influences on those rates may be very different in the developing world to those which hold in western industrialized countries.

Have caesarean rates stabilized?

It has been suggested that, although the trend for increased use of caesarean section continues, the rate of the escalation is beginning to slow down due to the increased use of VBAC, increased recognition of the imprecision of electronic fetal monitoring, greater public awareness and professional peer review activities (Marieskind, 1989). In the United States, by the late 1980s, there was some evidence to suggest that the caesarean rate had stabilized. From a rate of 24.1 per cent in 1986 it rose slightly to 24.4 per cent in 1987 and not very significantly again to 24.7 per cent in 1988. The rate of primary caesareans in 1988 of 17.5 per cent was almost identical to the rate of 17.4 per cent for the two previous years (Sanchez-Ramos et al., 1990). More recent evidence from North America suggests that the rate of caesareans may be decreasing as it was estimated to be 20.4 per cent in 1990 (Taffel et al., 1992). It has been suggested that the stabilization of caesarean rates is in large part due to the increased use of VBAC (Sanchez-Ramos et al., 1990) which increased from 9.8 per cent in 1987 to 12.6 per cent in 1988 representing the largest ever observed annual increase (Taffel et al., 1990). A study of caesarean rates in Norway, Sweden, Scotland and the United States found that rates were approaching stability in the four countries and were declining in Sweden (Notzen et al., 1994). However, although the caesarean section rate in Great Britain rose only slightly from 11 per cent in 1986 to 15.3 per cent in 1993, the rate of increase does not appear to have stabilized or reversed. During the period from 1985 to 1989, it rose by 0.2 per cent each year. From 1989 to 1992 the rate of increase was 0.3 per cent per annum (Francome et al., 1993), between 1992 and 1993 the rate of increase rose to its highest level ever at 2.0 per cent (Francome, 1994).

Reducing caesarean section rates

Vaginal Birth After Caesarean (VBAC)

The United States is the only region recorded to have reduced the number of caesareans in recent years. Between 1988 and 1989 the VBAC rate rose from 12.6 per cent to 18.5 per cent. This may have contributed to stemming the rise in the caesarean rates (Taffel et al., 1991). VBAC has also been cited as contributing to a reduction in the caesarean section rate in hospitals in other regions (Ziadeh and Sunna, 1995 [Jordan]).

Active Management of Labour (AML)

The aim of AML is to achieve delivery within 12 hours of the onset of labour (O'Driscoll et al., 1984). However, the onset of labour is difficult to assess and different practitioners take different indications. In addition, the assumption that individual women's labours will fit into a strictly defined timescale has been questioned (Savage, 1986; Axten, 1995). With AML, if the labour does not progress within the specified timescale the procedure is accelerated by the use of drugs (oxytocin intravenously). If the cervix fails to dilate at the rate of one centimetre per hour, artificial rupture of the membranes is performed.

It has been suggested that AML can reduce the incidence of caesarean section significantly without detriment to mother or child (Boylan et al., 1991). AML has been associated with a reduction in the caesarean section rate internationally (Maher et al. 1994 [Australia], Ziadeh and Sunna 1995 [Jordan]). After examination of the indications for performing caesareans, practitioners at one Glasgow hospital concluded that AML could be the most useful approach to reducing the caesarean section rate (Macara and Murphy, 1994). However, at one hospital known as 'the home of AML', the National Maternity Hospital in Dublin, the caesarean section rate has risen recently. The rise has been attributed to 'other indications' and not AML (How et al., 1995).

Audit and review

It appears that placing a close audit or monitoring programme on obstetric practice leading to caesarean section has an effect on the rates of caesarean delivery. During an audit of caesarean cases in the Scottish region of Dumfries and Galloway in 1986, the caesarean section rate dropped to 11.6 per cent from the 1985 rate of 15.8 per cent, an incredible decrease of 4.2 per cent (Urquhart et al., 1987). A New York State audit of obstetric practice in relation to caesarean section rates 1989–90 found a reversal of the section rate during the time of the audit. The downward trend was stronger in the reviewed rather than the non-reviewed hospitals (Dillon et al., 1992). Similarly a critical review of indications for caesarean section in one hospital department in Singapore found a reduction in the caesarean section rate for the period of review, particularly for cephalo-pelvic disproportion (Tay et al., 1992). Similar findings have been reported in a study from Australia with no detrimental effect on perinatal morbidity and mortality (Maher et al., 1994).

CHAPTER TEN

Indications for Caesarean Section

Indications for caesarean birth can be divided into two categories. First, medical indications, conditions of the pregnancy, the mother, baby or both that may mean that an abdominal delivery is advisable. However, within this category there are absolute and non-absolute (or relative) indications. Absolute indications for caesarean section include cephalopelvic disproportion and placenta praevia and usually mean that the baby cannot be born any other way. Relative indications for caesarean section include dystocia and fetal distress and rely on the individual case and/or the experience of the attending physician to decide whether a caesarean is necessary.

While it is hard to believe that caesarean sections would be performed for a reason other than medical necessity, there is a growing body of evidence to demonstrate the existence of 'social' or 'non-medical' indications for caesarean birth. Such indications are considered in the latter part of this chapter.

Medical indications for caesarean section in the late twentieth century

Dystocia

This term is used to describe a variety of different classifications of abnormal labour. Most commonly the term relates to complications regarding length of labour and fetal position or size but can be extended to include other problems occurring during the process of labour itself. Due to the vagueness in the definition of this diagnostic category it lends itself to individual interpretation and possibly over-use in situations where medical staff are unclear of how to proceed or are unwilling to proceed with a difficult labour.

Between 1970–78 dystocia was responsible for the largest contribution to the overall rise in the caesarean rate in the United States, accounting for as much as 30 per cent of the total. It appears that dystocia is increasingly being used as an indication for caesarean section. Between 1979 and 1980 the overall caesarean birth rate did not increase significantly in the United States but the distribution of caesarean sections by indication did change markedly. This change in distribution was primarily due to a shift in the use of dystocia as an indication from 24 per cent to 30 per cent of total caesareans

(Phillips et al., 1982). Therefore dystocia has come to be associated with increases in primary caesarean rates, and it is for this reason that the use of caesarean section for all cases of dystocia has been questioned (O'Driscoll et al., 1984) and the American National Institutes of Health's (NIH) report 'Cesarean Childbirth' recommended that this diagnostic category be thoroughly examined and reviewed (1981). In the 1990s dystocia is recognized as one of the major indications for caesarean section and its role in the world-wide increasing caesarean rate firmly established (How et al., 1995).

Fetal distress

Like dystocia, the term 'fetal distress' envelopes many conditions of the fetus.

> 'Fetal distress is a widely used but poorly defined term. This confusion of definition compounds the difficulty of making an accurate diagnosis and initiation of appropriate treatment.' (Parer and Livingston, 1990, p. 1421)

In general, fetal distress means that the baby is showing evidence of suffering from lack of oxygen (asphyxia) which could lead to brain damage. The commonest signs are that the baby becomes tired and moves less, it passes the contents of its bowel into the amniotic fluid, or that its heartbeat becomes abnormal. However, the vagueness of definition means that it is open to individual interpretation and thus can be misused in cases where the problem is unclear. The increased use of the diagnostic category of fetal distress over the past twenty years can be associated with the increases in the use of technology in the labour ward particularly as it relates to electronic fetal monitoring (EFM).

In Britain in the 1990s fetal distress is cited as indicating caesarean section in approximately one in five cases (see Chapter 12). The increasing trend in use of such non-specific terms has implications for the amount and type of information available to women being operated on. The use of categories such as dystocia and fetal distress without fuller explanation can be seen as one step in the disempowerment and alienation of women in the process of childbirth.

Cephalopelvic disproportion

(Pelvis too small or baby too large to exit via vaginal passage)
Historically the condition most often occurring under this heading was when the baby's head was too large to pass through the pelvic girdle. This may be due to the size or position of the baby or the size or shape of the mother's pelvis. More recently the term has been used to describe variations in the baby's position in the womb which may make the passage through the vagina difficult or dangerous. Although cephalopelvic disproportion is seen as an absolute indication for caesarean section (that is, there is no other option), the use of caesarean section for all cases is questionable. This category appears to have demonstrated the most substantial reduction in numbers in the 1990s (see Chapter 12).

Breech presentation

Breech presentation means that the fetus is positioned feet or bottom down for the time leading to delivery instead of the usual position of head first (vertex presentation). Breech presentations are associated with increased neonatal mortality and morbidity when compared to vertex presentation, irrespective of whether delivery is vaginal or by caesarean. Despite the fact that skilled practitioners can turn the fetus in utero (external cephalic version), there is an increasing trend for caesareans to be performed for breech presentation. In the United States the proportion of breech presentations delivered by caesarean rose from 11.6 per cent in 1970 to 60.1 per cent by 1978 (NIH, 1981). A similar trend was identifiable in this country. Statistics for the early 1980s in Britain show that about 40 per cent of breech presentations were delivered this way. However in a more recent calculation it emerged that 72 per cent of breech presentations in one health authority region in this country were by caesarean (Thorpe-Beeston et al., 1992).

An important question to consider here is whether the performing of caesarean sections improves outcome for breech presentations. Early data from New York City between 1967 and 1977 showed that for babies with a birth weight over 2500 grams, caesarean delivery of breech presentations indicated a neonatal mortality rate five-times better than the rate for vaginal delivery of breech presentation (NIH, 1981). Similarly researchers in Germany have suggested that caesarean section is preferable than vaginal birth for breech as this could possibly lead to an increased risk of cognitive retardation (Gotter and Kubinger, 1985). In the early 1990s a British study found better perinatal mortality rates for breech presentations delivered by caesarean than those delivered vaginally, 0.03 per cent compared to 0.83 per cent respectively. The researchers conluded that these data justified the wholesale performing of caesareans for breech presentation and that most mothers would opt for caesarean birth if informed of these statistics prior to delivery (Thorpe-Beeston et al., 1992).

Recent discussions have centred around the efficacy of external cephalic version (ECV) on infants presenting in breech in order to facilitate vaginal delivery and avoid caesarean section. Audit and research from the United States has demonstrated that ECV can reduce the caesarean section rate for breech presentation (Zhang et al., 1993; Calhoun et al., 1995). These results have been echoed in other parts of the world including the UK (Bewley et al., 1993; Cox, 1986), Australia (Goh et al., 1993; Foote, 1995) and Norway (Sand, 1993). Further, it has been demonstrated that EVC for breech presentation can be achieved without increasing perinatal morbidity or mortality (Foote, 1995).

Repeat caesareans and Vaginal Birth After Caesarean (VBAC)

The practice of repeat caesareans began in the early 1900s when the rationale behind it had a logical medical basis. At that time the vertical incision in the body of the uterus (classical) predominated and such incisions were prone to rupture particularly during the rigours of labour. However, the low segment transverse uterine incision in general use today is much less vulnerable to rupture and is associated with lower incidence of maternal and fetal morbidity and mortality. Thus the conviction that some obstetricians still carry today that 'once a caesarean, always a caesarean' appears to be more to do with tradition and a reluctance to change rather than being based on sound medical reasoning.

As primary caesarean rates rose, an inevitable rise in the number of repeat operations followed. This was evident primarily in the United States where repeat caesarean figures rose from 25.1 per cent in 1970 to 29.9 per cent in 1980 and 34.8 per cent in 1983. By 1985 this medical tradition had held for over 95 per cent of women for over a decade (Taffel et al., 1985). In Britain in the 1990s repeat caesareans are cited as indicators for operations in almost a quarter of cases (see Chapter 12), despite the radical change in procedure from vertical to low transverse incisions dating back to the 1930s. Evidence demonstrating the safety of VBAC has been available since the late 1960s, 'Rupture of lower segment is too uncommon to justify repetition of section for that reason alone' (McGarry, 1969, p.137). During the 1960s McGarry and his colleagues implemented a policy of attempting VBAC 'whenever it appeared safe'. This resulted in a successful vaginal delivery rate of 72.5 per cent of women with previous caesareans (1969). They concluded that elective repeat section after single previous lower segment caesareans may be required in less than 12 per cent of cases. In 1985 the WHO stated:

> 'There is no evidence that caesarean section is required after a previous transverse low segment caesarean section birth.' (p. 437)

In the year 1982–3 the success rate of VBAC at one Los Angeles centre was 82 per cent (Paul et al., 1985). A study of 2176 patients with one previous caesarean found that 90.8 per cent of women successfully delivered vaginally (Molloy et al., 1987). In Sweden the VBAC success rate over a ten year period involving 2036 women with previous caesareans was 92.2 per cent (Nielson et al., 1989). A study in one health region in this country found that 71 per cent of women with previous caesareans achieved vaginal delivery (Paterson and Saunders, 1991). It appears that over 70 per cent of women who have had one previous caesarean section will successfully deliver vaginally if allowed a trial of labour in a subsequent pregnancy and up to 85 per cent will be successful if the previous caesarean was for breech presentation (Paterson and Saunders, 1991). A success rate of up to 90 per cent was recorded in a recent survey in Great Britain (Savage and Francome, 1993).

As VBAC is increasingly being shown to be a viable and preferable alternative to repeat caesareans, there is also growing evidence to support trial of labour in patients with two or more prior caesareans as a safe and successful alternative to elective repeat caesarean sections (Hansell et al., 1990; Comerio et al., 1991; Cappa et al., 1991).

It has been demonstrated that VBAC is safe for the majority of women. VBAC mothers tend to have the same history and frequency of complications as mothers with previous vaginal deliveries (Placek and Taffel, 1988). Further, it could be suggested that repeat caesareans may actually be detrimental to women's health. Basing its comments on statistics gathered on caesareans being carried out in the United States, the NIH report (1981) stated that: 'a repeat cesarean carries two times the risk for maternal mortality of vaginal delivery' (p. 11). In a Swedish study significantly greater risks of major complications were found in repeat caesareans compared with primary caesareans (Nielsen and Hökegard, 1984).

The risk factor associated with repeat caesarean does not rest with the mother alone. In the States the Caesarean Birth Consensus Development Conference reported that at birth weights below 2501 grams, neonatal mortality is consistently higher for those born by caesarean compared with vaginal births. Therefore the evidence suggests that there is no advantage for mother or child of performing repeat caesareans (NIH, 1981).

The health risks to mothers and their babies from repeat caesareans, coupled with the fact that VBACs are cheaper than repeat caesareans in terms of hospital costs, means that the key to the use of VBAC in the future lies with public concern combined with an increased awareness by physicians, insurers and malpractice lawyers of the safety of VBAC.

However, the incidence of VBAC has only made small inroads against repeat caesarean section in the United States despite 1981 recommendations of the National Institutes of Health and 1982 'Guidelines for Vaginal Delivery after a Caesarean' issued by the College of Obstetricians and Gynaecologists stating that VBAC is safe for the majority of women with previous caesarean section (Shepperd McClain, 1990). A similar position has been established in this country (Walmsley and Hobbs, 1994). Thus there appears to be some reluctance among obstetricians to adopt a policy of VBAC as demonstrated in the overall rates. In 1980 the rate of VBAC in the United States among those women for whom it was feasible was 3.4 per cent (Taffel et al., 1985). The rate was 6.6 per cent by 1985 (Placek et al., 1987), 12.6 per cent in 1988 and rose to 20.4 per cent of women with previous caesareans in 1990 (Taffel et al., 1992).

It seems that it is reluctance on the part of many obstetricians and strict adherence to outdated medical traditions that is affecting decisions rather than the mother's current medical situation (Norman et al., 1993). Even when convinced of the intellectual rationale that VBAC is safe, it appears that situational pressures such as anxiety over legal liability, the inconvenience of a lengthy labour, peer pressure and general resistance to change may predispose obstetricians to retain outdated practices (Domnick Pierre et al., 1991). It certainly appears that whether or not women are offered the opportunity of VBAC is determined not only by their medical condition but also by the preferences of the obstetrician attending (Goldman et al., 1993).

However, some shift in obstetricians' attitude to VBAC is evident. The fact that the VBAC rate in the United States rose to over 20 per cent in 1990 may be an indication that VBAC is being more widely accepted and practiced. One health region in this country recently demonstrated that the practice of repeat caesareans may be in decline with 63 per cent of women with previous caesareans being allowed a trial of labour (Paterson and Saunders, 1991). A recent survey found that less than one in fifty British consultants follow a policy of repeat caesareans. The number in Scotland was one in twenty-four, which may account for the fact that the caesarean section rate was higher in Scotland than in England and Wales (Francome et al., 1993).

Therefore it appears that physicians' attitudes towards VBAC may be changing. The next hurdle is the attitudes of women as patients. There is some evidence to suggest that some women prefer elective caesarean sections to the potential discomfort of a trial of labour, especially after a previous experience with prolonged labour and eventual caesarean. Evidence, again from the States, has shown that in one hospital in New York offering a policy of VBAC for all eligible cases, 40 per cent of women declined the offer and opted for a repeat caesarean. It appears that fear of failed trial of labour and the convenience of a scheduled surgical delivery, coupled with negative attitudes of obstetricians towards a trial of labour, all contribute to women's choice of elective caesarean section (Shepperd McClain, 1990; Abitbol et al., 1993). Encouragement and counselling from hospital staff coupled with appropriate information on the feasibility of VBAC may be the key to changing women's attitudes about repeat caesareans. Hospitals with positive staff attitudes to VBAC and counselling programmes have demonstrated VBAC rates between 50 and 70 per cent of eligible women (Shepperd McClain, 1990; Penso, 1994). What this points to is that women need to be made aware of the feasibility of VBAC if they are to make informed choices.

Placenta praevia

This is a condition where the placenta is covering the neck of the womb (often causing bleeding) and indicating that a vaginal delivery would be problematic or impossible. Once the position of the placenta has been confirmed by ultrasound, a caesarean is usually arranged. This is done electively when the baby is mature or as an emergency if the bleeding is too heavy early in the pregnancy.

Multiple births

Twins account for about one in 80 births in the United Kingdom and the incidence of triplets is normally about one in 6,000. It is usually safe for twins and triplets to be born vaginally, yet many twins and most triplets are now born by caesarean. Quadruplets and higher order births are usually born by caesarean, but the evidence of this practice is scant (Francome et al., 1993). The caesarean rate has risen for twins, particularly the second twin as there is an increased chance that one of the babies will be breech or lie sideways in the uterus (transverse lie), but the rise in caesarean section for twin births does not seem justified by the evidence (Rydhström et al., 1990). However, caesarean rates for twin pregnancies present a minor part of overall caesarean statistics and do not make a significant contribution to overall caesarean rates.

Other maternal and fetal considerations

Many maternal and fetal conditions lead to a caesarean birth because of the need to deliver the infant as early as possible, such as cases of maternal diabetes, pregnancy-induced hypertension and erythroblastosis fetalis. However these conditions combined constitute a small contribution to the overall caesarean section rates.

Overall patterns

An examination of the major indications for caesarean section in the early 1980s revealed that while the overall caesarean rate for some countries were stabilizing, there was a shift in the distribution of caesareans for the various indications. The pattern of this change being towards the increasing use of dystocia and breech presentation as indications with a corresponding shift away from all other indications (Phillips et al., 1982). However, this shift was complete by the late 1980s. A study examining the indications for primary caesarean section found no decline in the top three indications for caesarean section: dystocia, breech presentation and fetal distress. Similarly, although the rates of vaginal birth after caesarean (VBAC) were increasing, they did not outweigh the effect of repeat caesareans on the rising caesarean rate (Myers and Gleicher, 1990). This picture has persisted to a large extent. My two studies of caesarean birth spanning a five year period (1991/2 and 1996) showed that repeat caesarean was the most commonly cited explanation. However, all the major indicators, including cephalopelvic disproportion, dystocia, fetal distress and breech presentation demonstrated some reduction in numbers (see Chapter 12).

Non medical variables affecting caesarean section rates

Declining birth rate

The declining birth rate in the industrial world since the 1960s has led to more emphasis on the outcome of pregnancy. It could be argued that the rise in caesarean section rates is a response to increased emphasis on the successful outcome of pregnancy. Given the declining birth rate and general faith in the medical profession, parental expectations have increased. Consultants continue to cite improved fetal outcomes as a reason for performing more caesareans despite evidence to show that there is no causal relationship between caesarean section rates above six per cent and better perinatal and neonatal outcomes (Francome et al., 1993). However, it appears that caesareans have become an acceptable approach in the attempt to improve fetal outcomes.

Hospitalization

Access to hospital resources has played a key role in increasing rates of caesarean section. Without the technical back-up and medical expertise that a well-equipped hospital offers, it is impossible to do major surgery, such as the caesarean, at an acceptable level of safety (Guillemin, 1981). What this means is that low risk women may receive excessive and unnecessary interventions simply because they give birth in hospital (Albers and Savitz, 1991). The fact that medical intervention is associated with availability of technological equipment means that women are more at risk of intervention if they give birth in hospital (Baruffi et al., 1990). Fullerton and Severino's 1992 study found that women in hospital were more likely to receive an interventionist style of labour and birth management, leading them to conclude that hospital care did not offer any advantage for women at lowest risk. This point is further demonstrated by the fact that in the United States, Birth Center (non-hospital) facilities have relatively fewer caesarean sections (Rooks et al., 1989). Therefore it appears that there is no evidence to suggest that hospitals are safer places for low-risk births yet hospitalization may put women at risk of increased levels of intervention.

Midwives and obstetricians

Related to the hospital/home debate is the midwives/obstetrician dichotomy. Evidence from the States has shown that women beginning their labour with midwives and/or in non-hospital settings attained considerably lower caesarean rates than women beginning their labours with physicians in hospitals (Sakala, 1993). The differences between midwife and obstetrician-managed patients appears to have an effect on the caesarean section rate. It has been demonstrated that even when controlling for risk factors known to increase the caesarean section rate, midwives attending births have lower rates of caesareans compared to births supervised by obstetricians (Macfarlane and Chamberlain, 1993; Rodin et al., 1993; Davis et al., 1994; Lydon-Rochelle, 1995). Obstetricians also tend to use epidural anaesthesia and oxytocin significantly more than midwives which increases the levels of caesarean section. Interestingly, no significant differences have been found in fetal outcomes between the two groups (Davis et al., 1994). It appears that the skills, attitudes and routines of midwives may explain part of this variation in intervention rates (Hemminki et al., 1992).

Technological management of labour

Evidence suggests that the unregulated introduction and use of technology can unduly increase intervention rates. A year-long study in 1981 demonstrated the startling effects of the introduction of a perinatology service to one hospital in the United States. The caesarean section rate increased from 14.3 per cent to 18.5 per cent. Furthermore, the implementation of careful monitoring and review procedures produced a reversal of the caesarean rate to its former level (Lomas and Enkin, 1989).

The rate of intervention in childbirth is accelerated by an emphasis on time scales combined with a rigid adherence of the three stages of labour. It has been suggested that one intervention leads to another and there is evidence to support this view. This contention is not new. Almost twenty years ago Ann Cartwright found that women who were induced more often had assisted deliveries (1979). Epidural anaesthesia has been associated with increased incidence of caesarean birth (Eakes, 1990; Thorp et al., 1990; Morton et al., 1994). Thus treatments early in labour often culminate in the ultimate intervention, caesarean section (see Figure 10.1).

What this spiral of events means is that medical students, doctors and midwives in training do not see as many normal labours as they need to in order to understand the individual pattern and differences between women, instead of relying on estimates of an average range of women in labour (Savage, 1986). This point is taken a step further by midwife Sally Inch who suggests that the emphasis on intervention in childbirth, and thus the control of delivery by obstetricians, will lead to a deskilling of midwives and doctors leaving them unable to deal with anything other than a singleton, vertex delivery, as all else will be delivered abdominally (1986). This view is supported by the fact that a 1984 study found that the incidence of caesarean birth for second twins (following vaginal delivery of the first) rose from 0.33 per cent between 1973 and 1982

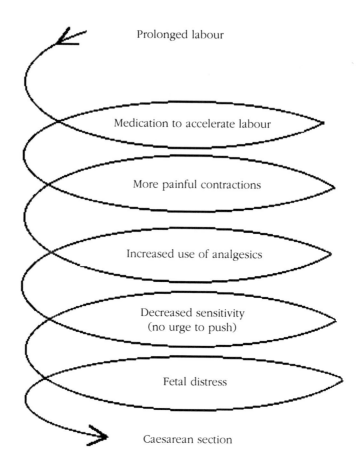

Prolonged labour

Medication to accelerate labour

More painful contractions

Increased use of analgesics

Decreased sensitivity
(no urge to push)

Fetal distress

Caesarean section

Fig. 10.1: Technological management of labour spiral

to seven per cent by the mid 1980s, a finding that the researchers put down to declining obstetric skills and experience (Olofsson and Rydhström, 1985). Further, the use of fetal monitoring, poorly understood when it was first introduced, has lead to a devaluation of the skills and 'art' of midwifery (Savage, 1986). On a similar theme Kitzenger suggested that in cases where the baby is lying in a difficult position, obstetricians in the past would have attempted to correct the position by external version, wheras the tendency now is to deliver the baby by caesarean section rather than attempting to turn the baby. The result of this is that obstetricians have been deskilled and no longer know how to perform external version (Kitzenger, 1980).

Anxiety and fear of litigation
Anxiety among the medical profession is an underlying factor in the rise in intervention rates in childbirth generally. A recent factor which has increased anxiety among health care professionals in this country is the fear of litigation. If there are problems associated with the birth then the doctor can be sued. Whereas if a caesarean is carried out, any resulting problems (including the death of the mother) are considered to be a normal

risk of the operation. 'High risk', in terms of childbirth, it has been suggested, has come to mean the likelihood of being sued rather than encountering complications during delivery (Inlander, 1990). This is an important factor in the high caesarean rate in the United States where not only can private patients sue for damage caused to infants during birth but also the concept of 'wrongful life' makes it possible for the damaged survivor of a problematic birth to gain recompense for a costly existence (Guillemin, 1981). Patients in the United States must sue the hospital and it is the hospital that has to pay if a ruling is made in favour of the patient. It is therefore argued that defensive medicine is responsible for the high caesarean section rate in private practice.

In the past, fear of malpractice suits was the most frequent reason for the increase in the caesarean section rate given by physicians in surveys in both the United States (Marieskind, 1989) and in the United Kingdom (Boyd and Francome, 1986). Further evidence suggests that this trend is continuing to have an effect on caesarean rates in this country. In 1992 almost half (46.8 per cent) of doctors surveyed said that the caesarean rates were rising in Britain because of fear of litigation (Francome et al., 1993). By 1993 that proportion had risen considerably (Francome, 1994).

According to Capsticks, a law firm specializing in medical litigation, every year since 1983 about one in 2,500 births has been followed by legal action. But claims had nearly doubled by the early 1990s, especially since changes in the procedures for claiming legal aid were instituted in 1990 (Macnair, 1992). Thus fear of litigation has pushed up the caesarean section rate. It has been suggested that doctors in general, and obstetricians in particular, are responsible for their own downfall. By inculcating among the general public the image of super-heroes who can rescue women from their sufferings and come up with a perfect baby every time, it has become virtually impossible for the average person to come to terms with the fact that doctors can be fallible (Ranjan, 1993). What this means is that the public have come to expect remarkable achievements and perfect results every time. It is therefore assumed that the obstetrician is negligent if something goes wrong.

Obstetrician Wendy Savage states that the stress of working in an environment where errors of judgement made in good faith are treated as 'crimes' and a climate where perfection is assumed to be a realistic possibility despite human error, poor management systems and a declining service over which doctors and midwives have no real control, increases anxiety levels. This problem is exacerbated by the fact that women are likely to see a range of different professionals who may offer her differing opinions or explain things in a way that the woman finds difficult to understand because they do not know her. Savage suggests, however, that when the woman knows the professionals who are caring for her, and, because the relationship is based on mutual trust, if something does go wrong the woman does not usually blame her midwife or doctor (1986). This point is reiterated by Ranjan who suggests that the majority of litigation cases against doctors reflect poor communication and rapport between patient and clinician either before, during or after the event (1993).

The tide of rising caesarean rates due to fear of litigation could be reversed by the introduction of no fault compensation for birth injuries, thereby acknowledging that parents of children damaged at birth need support regardless of allocation of blame.

This system has worked well in New Zealand since 1974 whereby doctors receive immunity from court action for negligence if a problem occurs in the course of treating a patient. Yet if the standard of medical treatment falls below what is acceptable, the doctor can still be sued (Ranjan, 1993). What this means is that individuals can receive compensation for problems occurring during medical treatment when the decisions for the particular treatment were taken in good faith. Doctors, therefore, do not need to practice defensive medicine and patients receive compensation commensurate with the degree of injury suffered.

One of the most disturbing factors associated with the practice of caesareans based on fear of litigation is that the women involved are not being given the correct information in terms of the reasons for performing the operation. Obstetricians are not likely to inform a woman that they are about to carry out a caesarean in order to cover themselves in the event of something going wrong with the birth.

Age of mother as a 'high risk' factor

Maternal age has always been a consideration in decisions on whether or not to perform a caesarean. The older the mother is, the more likely she is to be delivered by caesarean. Evidence from Europe and the Americas has demonstrated a clear link between maternal age and caesarean section rates. It appears that women in the higher age categories (that is, over 30 years of age) are at high risk of delivering by caesarean section (Bertollini et al., 1992; Zahniser et al., 1992; Adashek et al., 1993; Peipert and Bracken, 1993).

What seems to be happening is that more and more women are included in this high risk category and there are no guidelines for the classification of age as a risk factor. Thus the designation of women to this category has varied from early classifications of women in their forties to the more recent inclusion of women in their late twenties. This rising caesarean rate among younger mothers has given additional momentum to the rising caesarean rate in general, not only because more younger women are being operated on, but also because a significant proportion of subsequent deliveries will be by caesarean.

Changes in diagnostic practices and procedures

Increases in the number of caesarean sections being performed may be in part due to the increased diagnosis of fetal distress in labour (NIH, 1981; Inch, 1985). A further reason for the increase in the caesarean rate involves major changes in the obstetrical management of breech presentation (NIH, 1981; Taffel et al., 1985). Both are now cited as major indicators for caesarean section in obstetric literature.

Electronic fetal monitoring (EFM)

Evidence linking EFM with higher caesarean rates is unequivocal (McCusker et al., 1988). When all factors except the use of EFM are controlled, the caesarean section rate almost doubles as a result of using EFM (Inch, 1985). The use of EFM has also been linked with the increasing frequency of diagnosis of fetal distress (NIH, 1981). In a study of British consultants' views on the rising caesarean rate, one in eighteen mentioned the misreading of EFM as a reason for the increase in rates. Some of the respondents were positive about the use of EFM: 'monitoring enables us to identify babies at risk'. Others were less confident about the benefits of EFM and felt that the rising caesarean rates were due to: 'misinterpretation of fetal monitoring results' or 'too much monitoring and too little facts' (Francome et al., 1993, p. 131). It is therefore reasonable to assume that the rising caesarean rate is to some extent the result of the increased use of EFM.

Finance

Financial factors also lead to increases in the caesarean section rate and may act against the best care being given to pregnant women. Such considerations have had a role to play in the high caesarean section rates in the United States. The differing caesarean section rates for women of differing socio-economic status can be interpreted as relating to differing financial incentives for physicians. Where payment is involved in health care it is more lucrative for the doctor to perform a caesarean as it can be done in a shorter time than a vaginal delivery and she/he will be paid more (Francome, 1990). Fees for caesarean birth are often higher than those for vaginal delivery, charges for caesarean operations in the United States can be more than double those for uncomplicated vaginal deliveries and there is evidence to suggest that financial considerations do play a part in physicians' decisions on whether or not to perform a caesarean (Guillemin, 1981; Janowitz et al., 1984). Wealthier, insured groups of the population suffer higher rates of caesarean section than their lower socio-economic counterparts (Stafford, 1991; Stafford et al., 1993; Zahniser et al., 1992; Keeler and Brodie, 1993). This suggests that profit has become a valid indicator for caesarean section rather than medical need or concern for the women involved. It also means that women who are more likely to experience complications in pregnancy such as low birth weight infants and perinatal mortality, that is, women in the lower socio-economic groups, are least likely to have a caesarean (Shearer, 1993).

However, it has been suggested that the direct effect of financial considerations on caesarean section rates should not be overestimated. In some cases the difference between fees for caesareans and for vaginal deliveries are not that great and may actually have been removed altogether. Also, the proportion of the fees which translates into income for the physician is likely to be negligible and therefore will not have a large effect on the decision to perform the operation. However, it has been suggested that the indirect relationship between the financial income from operative birth as opposed to vaginal delivery is more likely to emerge from the physicians' ability to control the time and duration of the delivery with caesarean section which is not afforded by spontaneous labour and delivery (Lomas and Enkin, 1989).

But how does this relate to an increasing caesarean rate in National Health Service (NHS) hospitals? In an atmosphere of financial constraints on health services, with hospitals having to ration resources and manage tight budgets, it is not unreasonable to expect that highly technological, expensive equipment, along with highly trained personnel, need to be seen to be efficient, effective and, more importantly, over-used in order to justify their existence. Such considerations could inadvertently affect the caesarean section rate.

Medical convenience

There is evidence to suggest that medical interventions in childbirth, including caesarean section, are carried out for reasons of convenience for the medical practitioners rather than for the medical need of the woman concerned. More sections are performed during the day than at night and during the week rather than at the weekend (Macfarlane, 1984; Bertollini et al., 1992). Cartwright's 1979 study showed that elective caesareans were more likely to occur on Mondays and relatively few were performed at weekends. One respondent in a US study of women who had had caesareans said:

> 'Sometime during the day the nurses had told us it was my doctor's birthday and that he was having a party that night. As they were taking me to the delivery room they made my husband wait in the hall. While he was waiting there he heard my doctor on the 'phone say, "You go ahead without me to the party; I'll be there in 45 minutes".' (Perez, 1989, p. 132)

Some procedures and practices may by utilized in hospital for practitioner convenience rather than patient need. For example, the supine position in labour is more convenient for practitioners and the use of machinery but is not the most efficient for the progress of labour and may lead to dystocia and caesarean birth (Freda, 1994). Mavis Kirkham, from her experience of working as a midwife, implies that pain relief is given to women during labour to relieve the discomfort of the medical staff present (1986). This raises the question of whether other interventions, and even surgery, are performed for the same reason. In a letter to *The Lancet*, Smith, whilst defending the caesarean section rate stated: 'No woman these days has a labour of over fifteen hours without her... becoming agitated, let alone the midwife and junior medical staff' (1990). The implication here is that caesareans are performed for the ease/comfort of the medical practitioners rather than being dependent on the medical needs of women having babies.

The argument that caesareans are being performed for practitioner convenience rather than medical necessity is furthered by the fact that the incidence of respiratory distress syndrome is less among infants whose mothers are allowed to go into labour prior to the caesarean being performed than those whose mothers are operated on before the onset of labour (Cohen and Carson, 1985; Lagercrantz and Slotkin, 1986). Yet still it is the norm to perform elective caesareans before the onset of spontaneous labour. The implication here is that it is more convenient for the physician, hospital and patient for a pre-planned elective operation rather than waiting for labour to begin, even though the evidence suggests that this is better for the infant. It could therefore be suggested that caesareans are contemplated for reasons of convenience as doctors and hospital staff will know exactly when the baby is to be born and roughly how long it will take rather than waiting for the unpredictable timing and duration of spontaneous labour.

Staffing

The issue of 'staffing' has been raised by consultants as a problem and a reason for the increase in the caesarean section rate either because less experienced junior doctors are staffing labour wards or because the consultants' workloads have increased (Francome et al., 1993). This may well be the case.

'Unfortunately, much of the labour ward obstetrics is in the hands of registrars and other relatively junior staff at present. Consultants may be contacted about a doubtful case by telephone, but often the easier answer is tell the registrar to carry on with a section.' (Chamberlain, 1993, p. 403)

Similarly, evidence suggests that a higher ratio of women to consultants is associated with a higher caesarean section rate (Health Committee, 1992). This will inevitably have an effect on the caesarean section rate as services are scrutinized for efficiency and consultants' workloads are increased in the name of rationalization.

Consultants: preference and prestige

The differential rates of caesarean section between countries, regions, hospitals and individual consultants has been blamed on the failure to establish basic principles regarding technological intervention in childbirth. Some commentators have suggested that this failure has led to diverse practices in obstetrics and to women's encounters with maternity services being such a 'pot luck affair' (Hughes and Parker, 1986, p. 62). A study of physicians' individual caesarean rates in one North American hospital demonstrated a range from 4.3 per cent to 12.3 per cent of deliveries (DeMott and Sandmire, 1992). It has also been suggested that practicing surgery is a way by which obstetricians are able to acquire a certain amount of kudos, 'A peculiar distinction of obstetrics is its dual identity as a surgical speciality' (Guillemin, 1981, p. 16).

It appears that individual physician characteristics do influence caesarean section rates significantly, including factors such as place of medical education and country of medical training (Tussing and Wojtowycz, 1993).

Gender of the physician

One study found that female physicians have slightly lower caesarean section rates than their male counterparts (Tussing and Wojtowycz, 1993). It may be that female physicians are more reluctant to operate on other women to extract an infant, as they may have more empathy with the importance that vaginal delivery has for women. However, a survey in this country found no correlation between the sex of the obstetrician and individual caesarean section rates (Savage and Francome, 1993) (see Chapter eight for a more detailed account of the influence of gender on the doctor-patient relationship).

The cost of caesareans

The continuing rise in caesareans raises important implications for health care costs and medical providers. The medical cost of delivery by caesarean is higher than that of vaginal delivery (NIH, 1981). The average length of hospital stay for caesarean patients is almost double that of vaginal deliveries (Taffel et al., 1985), whereas the length of hospital stay for VBAC mothers is comparable to other vaginal deliveries (Placek and Taffel, 1988). In the United States it was estimated that if the 500,000 repeat caesareans had been VBAC, surgical fees and costs for 1.2 million days of hospital stay would have been averted between 1980 and 1985 (Placek and Taffel, 1988). Further, it has been estimated that approximately half the caesareans performed in the United States are unnecessary, resulting in an avoidable expense of over $1 billion each year (Shearer, 1993).

In Britain the rising cost of maternity services is partly the result of increased intervention in childbirth including caesarean section. Intervention increases the demand for expensive paediatric and anaesthetic facilities. The wider use of elective caesareans increases the demand for biochemical and ultrasound facilities for assessment of gestational age. It has been estimated that a woman delivered by caesarean section is likely to cost the NHS at least £1000 more than if she had a vaginal delivery. Therefore if the caesarean rate was reduced by only one per cent it would save the Health Service £7,000,000 a year (Savage and Francome, 1993). Lomas and Enkin state that:

> 'An emerging cost-consciousness makes it less and less acceptable to spend resources on interventions that are being used at rates far in excess of what can be considered appropriate, or even "good medicine".' (Lomas and Enkin, 1989, p. 1193)

In times of scarce resourcing for the health services, it is inappropriate to channel so much money into the increasing use of interventionist techniques which are of questionable value.

CHAPTER ELEVEN

The Effects of Caesarean Section

Effects of caesarean section on the mother

Caesareans affect women differently to vaginal deliveries. The evidence suggests that women who have caesarean births suffer more negative effects, both psychologically and physiologically. The negative effects of caesarean sections are compounded by such things as having emergency operations as opposed to elective ones, the type of anaesthetic used for the operation, whether a partner/birth companion was allowed to be present for the birth, and how prepared the woman was for the operation in terms of the amount of information available to her about caesarean birth.

Emergency versus elective caesareans

Studies have shown that women who have emergency operations have less positive perceptions of the delivery than women who have either vaginal or elective caesarean deliveries (Cranley et al., 1983; Fawcett et al., 1992; Francome et al., 1993; Reichert et al., 1993) and that they report significantly more distress regarding the physical sensations associated with the birth (Fawcett et al., 1992). Women who have unplanned caesareans often feel that they have failed because they could not give birth vaginally and have, in some circumstances, even blamed their babies for the long, painful, and unproductive labours that resulted in operative deliveries, postpartum pain and emotional distress (Marut and Mercer, 1979; Affonso and Stichler, 1980). These findings suggest that the unexpected nature of the unplanned caesarean delivery may have more influence on the woman's feelings about her birth experience than the caesarean delivery per se. This is probably because in the emergency situation there may not be time for the procedure to be explained to the woman or for the medical practitioners to keep the woman fully informed of all that is happening to her. However, when the caesarean is elective the woman has time to acquire the knowledge and information she will need to deal appropriately with the operation. She will have time to read about caesarean birth and to discuss any queries with health professionals which should enable her to come to terms with what is about to happen and thereby avoid the feelings of complete disappointment that many caesarean patients feel. In cases of emergency caesarean, women do not have the luxury of time. One study found that almost half the women having emergency caesareans had two hours or less to prepare themselves for the operation. The researchers concluded that this was too short a time for the women to grasp the significance of what was happening and therefore deal with the situation appropriately (Affonso and Stichler, 1980). Similarly other studies have recorded negative responses from unplanned caesareans (Marut and Mercer, 1979; Fawcett, 1981; Francome et al., 1993; see also pp. 144–145).

Emergency caesareans also appear to carry a higher risk of morbidity and mortality for women, although this is to some extent due to the conditions necessitating the emergency operation rather than the surgery per se. In a study of the surgical complications of caesarean section, Nielsen and Hökegürd found that the major complications associated with all procedures all occurred in emergency operations. For example, blood transfusions were used five times more often in emergency operations than elective caesareans. Correspondingly all complications associated with elective procedures were minor ones (1984). Emergency caesareans are also more risky in terms of death to the mother. All maternal deaths (except one) following caesarean section in Sweden between 1973 and 1979 occurred after an emergency operation (Moldin et al., 1984). In the UK deaths following caesarean delivery still occur more frequently following emergency operations. However, the latest official data available shows a decline in the number of deaths following unplanned emergency operations (DoH, 1991 and 1994).

Type of anaesthetic

The type of anaesthetic used for the operation is also important. Caesarean delivered women who have had regional anaesthesia tend to have a more positive perception of the birth experience than those who have general anaesthesia (Marut and Mercer, 1979; Cranley et al., 1983; Fawcett et al., 1992; Francome et al., 1993; Reichert et al., 1993). This is possibly because women who have regional anaesthetic remain conscious throughout the operation and are therefore able to feel as though they are taking part in the birth process. Participation in the decision-making process is the most important component indicated by women in terms of their satisfaction with medical care (Seguin et al., 1989). Epidural anaesthetic makes the process easier for mothers particularly in the early postnatal period as they can benefit from early contact with their newborn babies and it leaves them free to respond to their babies needs and feel more confident in their abilities to care for their infants (Trowell, 1986; Francome et al., 1993). The use of regional anaesthesia has also been shown to have a less negative effect on the mother-infant relationship (Gottlieb and Barrett, 1986).

Mothers having epidural anaesthesia appear to have a better experience all round. Not only are they better informed, and thus prepared, awake for the birth of their babies and often have their partners present, they suffer less after-effects. They usually get out of bed earlier than women who have had general anaesthesia, they feed their babies sooner, report less depression and tiredness in the postpartum period, as well as having a lower incidence of a wide range of complications such as infection (Morgan et al., 1984).

There appears to be a significant difference in post-operative morbidity according to the type of anaesthetic used for the caesarean operation (Morgan et al., 1984). In a review of relevant studies on the negative effects of caesarean section, Oakley and Richards (1990) found that mothers who had been given general anaesthetic for their operations experienced more marked effects than women having epidurals. A French survey found that mothers having general anaesthetic experienced longer-lasting consequences, such as tiredness, and experienced more difficulties taking care of their babies (Lelong and Kaminski, 1987). Not surprisingly, more women feel tired and depressed following general anaesthesia for caesareans than those who have epidurals (Morgan et al., 1984).

Furthermore, general anaesthesia carries with it the risk of death associated with all major surgical procedures (Chalmers and Richards, 1977). The Department of Health reports on maternal deaths in the United Kingdom highlight the risks. Between 1976 and 1978, 57 per cent of maternal deaths in England and Wales were associated with the use of general anaesthesia for emergency caesarean sections (DHSS, 1982). Of the eight women whose deaths were directly related to anaesthesia administered during delivery between 1985 and 1987, seven women were given the anaesthesia for caesarean operations (DoH, 1991). In the triennium 1988 to 1990 four out of five deaths related to anaesthesia were caesarean patients (DoH, 1994).

On the whole, it appears that there is an association between type of anaesthesia used for the caesarean operation and the woman's attitude towards the delivery. Ninety three per cent of Sargent and Stark's sample said that being in control was important to them. The association between local anaesthesia and maintaining control was evident (1989). General anaesthesia tends to be associated with more negative perceptions. This is probably because women who have general anaesthesia for their caesarean operations are not able to participate in the birth of their children and often feel deprived of the experience and the memories that are associated with it. It appears that 'being awake' for the birth represents 'participation' in the delivery for many women (Sargent and Stark, 1989). Opportunity to participate in the decision-making process and, more importantly, to participate in the delivery of the baby are critical elements in perceptions of caesarean childbirth (Sargent and Stark, 1987).

> 'I was pleased to be able to have this operation under epidural rather than a general anaesthetic. Thus allowing me to see the baby earlier and be part of the birth process.' (Francome et al., 1993, p. 103)

Thus the evidence shows that the combination of emergency operations and general anaesthesia offer the greatest risk to women in terms of post-operative morbidity, and more importantly, maternal mortality.

'MISSING PIECES'

A major effect of general anaesthesia is that women are unable to recall the birth experience and therefore do not feel as though they have participated in it. It has been suggested that this lack of recollection is responsible for general negative feeling towards the birth process (Sargent and Stark, 1987; Francome et al., 1993). In Sargent and Stark's study a significant proportion of their sample (41 per cent) reported that some significant aspect of the birth experience was 'missing'. One of their respondents said: 'I feel I missed the whole experience'. Another stated: 'when I awoke it was over'. Such experiences lead to feelings of doubt in the women concerned. One said: 'How do I know she's mine? I didn't see her come out' (1987, p. 1272). Similar experiences are evident in this country: 'With having a general, I feel I missed out on the first moments' (Francome et al., 1993, p. 99).

It has also been suggested that people are more able to cope with stressful experiences if they have been witness to events as they unfold (Huntingford, 1985). If this is the case, then the experience of women undergoing caesarean section could be improved if they are awake for the operation. Given the negative after-effects associated with general anaesthesia, such as maternal feelings of dissatisfaction with the delivery, increased incidence of morbidity and the risk of mortality, there must surely be an argument for the use of regional anaesthesia in all possible cases.

Having a partner/birth companion present for the birth

The benefits of having a friend or partner present for the birth are obvious. Not only are they able to offer direct support to the mother but they are also able to act as mediator between the woman and the medical staff and assist in negotiations about what may happen. At a time when the woman is feeling particulary anxious and vulnerable, it is essential that she has someone who knows her well with her to act as advocate. Furthermore, the woman's disappointment at missing out on the birth of her child, as when general anaesthetic is used, may be reduced if her friend or partner is able to give her an account of the birth which otherwise she may not have. A partner's description of the birth with details that medical attendants may consider trivial can do a lot to make up for what the mother has missed (Huntingford, 1985). Studies looking at women's experiences of caesarean section have shown that women express much greater satisfaction with the operation when they have been able to have their partner present for the birth (Marut and Mercer, 1979; Fawcett, 1981; Cranley et al., 1983; Cain et al., 1984; May and Sollidd, 1984; Francome et al., 1993). Furthermore, the presence of the partner in the operating room tends to improve the post-operative behavioural response of both parents (NIH, 1981).

HOSPITAL/DOCTOR POLICY

Whether or not the partner/birth companion is allowed to be present for a caesarean is very much reliant on the personal preference of the doctor attending the birth. A survey of obstetricians found that almost half (47.8 per cent) of consultants said that they would allow a birth companion to be present for a caesarean. A similar number said that they would allow it 'sometimes'. Only 3.7 per cent said that partners/birth companions were not invited into the operating theatre for abdominal deliveries. The crucial factor in whether or not consultants allow a partner/birth companion to be present, on the whole, was the use of general anaesthesia (Francome et al., 1993). Thus at a time when great stress is being placed on the desirability of 'sharing' the birth experience, some couples may experience considerable stress and disappointment if the partner is excluded.

ARE PARTNERS A NUISANCE IN THE OPERATING THEATRE?

Some doctors state that it is inconvenient for partners to be present during a caesarean as the serious nature of the operation means that the presence of an extra person in the theatre may present some kind of a risk. However, it appears that the partner's presence in the operating theatre does not constitute a major problem or risk (NIH, 1981). Fears about the adverse effect of partners being present during surgery in terms of, for example, risks of infection, the partner not being able to cope with what is happening and becoming an extra burden on the medical staff, lack of space and an increase in the number of malpractice suits have never been proved (Hillan, 1991). Huntingford states that in his experience as a Consultant Obstetrician, there is no anticipated complication or even tragedy at birth which justifies exclusion of the partner:

> 'In the end it is usually easier to accept and come to terms with what happens if you have been a witness to events as they unfold, rather than if bad news is conveyed to you by a stranger afterwards.' (Huntingford, 1985, p. 132)

What this points to, once again, is that it is better for the woman and her partner/birth companion if regional anaesthesia is used instead of general. The use of general anaesthetic tends to mean the exclusion of all but the patient and medical staff from the birth in some hospitals.

Psychological effects

The evidence from existing studies suggests that women may be less satisfied following caesarean birth than those who deliver vaginally, and that this dissatisfaction may contribute to feelings of depression, disappointment, guilt, lower self-esteem and could possibly have long term effects on the mother-child relationship. Women who have delivered by caesarean section have been observed to experience intense post-operative anxiety, extreme disappointment and a sense of inadequacy and failure (Cohen, 1977; Affonso and Stichler, 1980; Francome et al., 1993).

DISAPPOINTMENT, GUILT AND DEPRESSION

Depression is a commonly accepted consequence of major surgery yet the assumption is not made about caesarean section. However, it has been suggested that there is a clear relationship between technologically managed delivery generally and postnatal depression (Oakley, 1980), but more specifically, there is a relationship between caesarean section and depression postnatally (MacArthur et al., 1991; Hannah et al., 1992). Anxiety and depression in relation to motherhood is predominantly seen as reflecting the feminine psyche and not as rational concomitants of surgical experiences (Oakley, 1980). Many of the psychological consequences of surgery in general will also apply to caesarean section including emotional relief or elation at having survived the operation, worry about the mutilating effects of the surgery on the body and a protracted period of physical and psychological discomfort.

It is often the case that any sign of negative emotion from the caesarean mother is put down to the 'baby blues' or 'feeling a bit weepy' after the birth and therefore not usually associated with the surgery that the woman has undergone. Yet the caesarean patient is expected to cope, not only with these feelings with little or no support and understanding, but also with the demands of a newborn baby, thereby engaging in activities which would not normally be expected of patients who have had major abdominal surgery. This will inevitably exacerbate any feelings of depression as the woman will not be able to cope with her baby in the way that she had expected to. Unless women have a previous history of difficult labour, previous caesareans or are alerted during antenatal check-ups that a caesarean may be necessary, they will not usually seriously consider that they could need a section. They are therefore more disappointed when the outcome does not meet their expectations and are likely to suffer more in terms of depression because of this. Further, it has been suggested that caesarean section increases the incidence of more serious depression and anxiety postnatally in some mothers (Trowell, 1986). Caesarean mothers have also been shown to report less satisfaction with the birth experience than those who delivered vaginally (Marut and Mercer, 1979; Cranley et al., 1983; Kearney et al., 1990).

In addition to these feelings the obstetric patient may experience a sense of loss and even failure at not being able to deliver normally. There is evidence to suggest that caesarean mothers feel disappointment or anger at being 'cheated' of a vaginal delivery (see pp. 141–42) which leads to feelings of depression, guilt and lack of self-esteem (Cox and Smith, 1982; Reichert et al., 1993). 'You can't class caesarean as giving birth, I don't feel as if I have really had a baby.' (Francome et al., 1993, p. 108). Furthermore, women are subjected to the sometimes damaging or depressing effect of not being able to control what happens during the delivery (Richards, 1983). One woman's account of her reactions when she found out that she would need a caesarean highlights this point:

> 'I've known for two days that I'd have to have a Caesarean section. My baby is a breech presentation and my pelvis too small for a vaginal delivery. I feel like a freak – not a "real" woman – I can't even be delivered "normally". I shall never know the experience of childbirth. I shall never be able to say, "Oh it wasn't that bad". I'll never know what it feels like to push the baby I've carried inside me into the world.' (Dean, 1986, p. 70)

Women have reported feelings of disappointment and guilt about not being able to 'mother' the newborn immediately after delivery. In Fawcett and Burritt's study, one woman stated that she felt guilty that she was not interested in the baby for a day, and that she was concerned that lack of early bonding would have lasting negative effects on her relationship with her infant (1985). More recent data from this country has highlighted this point (see Chapters 12 and 13).

LONG TERM PSYCHOLOGICAL EFFECTS

A woman's feelings about her childbearing experience may influence her feelings about, and performance of, her perceived maternal role. New mothers frequently regard the birth experience as a nodal event that can colour the rest of their lives (Marut and Mercer, 1979). Negative feelings about the birth may therefore have a negative impact on family life. What is clear is that mothers delivered by caesarean section need time to recover physically and need extra support emotionally. Many women and their families handle this satisfactorily. But it has been suggested that for many it is a struggle and for a number of them the operation leaves them pre-occupied and unresponsive to their baby so that their perception of the child as difficult can persist (Trowell, 1986).

Evidence from studies investigating the long-term effects of caesarean birth, while limited in scope, raise a number of important issues. Caesarean mothers tend to handle their infants significantly less in the immediate postpartum period (Tulman, 1986) and experience more ambivalence towards their babies (Affonso and Stichler, 1980). In a study comparing 50 low risk primigravidae delivered by caesarean section with a matched control group of 50 primigravidae delivered vaginally, Edith Hillan found that six months after the delivery, more of the emergency caesarean women were adamant that they would never have another baby and the majority stated that their decision was a direct result of their labour and delivery experiences. In the control group the decision to have no more children was found to be unrelated to labour and birth experiences (1992).

Similarly, a study in France found that four years after delivery, caesarean birth had long-term effects on mothers' physical and psychological states. Caesarean women had fewer children, experienced more difficulties conceiving and reported fatigue more frequently (Garel et al., 1990).

INCONCLUSIVE EVIDENCE ON PSYCHOLOGICAL EFFECTS
Evidence on the negative effects of caesarean section is not conclusive and some studies have suggested that mothers having caesarean birth are not significantly different on levels of depression than those delivering vaginally (Bradley, 1983; Culp and Osofsky, 1989; Sargent and Stark, 1987) and that many women perceive the operation to be a positive experience (Sargent and Stark, 1987). Further, it has been suggested that the most important dimension of birth to the women involved is a healthy baby and not the delivery process (Sargent and Stark, 1987).

One study comparing the effects of caesarean delivery with vaginal births found that the mothers and fathers experiencing caesarean births were not significantly different on levels of depression or marital adjustment and there were no significant differences in the mother-infant behaviour during the feedings observed. The authors suggested that these results support the theory that mothers respond to their babies' behavioural repertoire and not to the mode of delivery (Culp and Osofsky, 1989).

What is more, it has been suggested that caesarean parents see their children in a more positive light or react more positively to them during the first year, and that these early parental perceptions and reactions persist. Explanations for this offered by the authors of this study centre around the caesarean child being perceived as more valuable or 'precious' to its parents. For example, caesarean children are more costly (where direct payment for medical care is involved). Also, caesareans are perceived to be more dangerous and are more debilitating to the mother in the short term. Caesarean parents, having suffered these negative concomitants of caesarean birth, could therefore place a higher value on their infant as a consequence. However, the authors do concede that the circumstances surrounding the birth of a child may affect family process over lengthy periods of time (Entwisle and Alexander, 1987).

Researching into the differences in psychological adjustment and satisfaction between women who delivered vaginally and those delivered by caesarean section, Padawer et al. found that, although there were significant differences in levels of satisfaction, (caesarean mothers reporting less satisfaction with the delivery and childbirth experience than the vaginal birth mothers) caesarean mothers were not more depressed, anxious or less confident in their mothering abilities than the women who delivered vaginally, and no differences were found between the groups on psychological adjustment. There were no indications of decreased mental health or need for clinical intervention among the women in the caesarean group (1988). However this study controlled many of the factors associated with caesarean birth that tend to lead to women experiencing detrimental effects from the operation. Factors such as participation in childbirth classes, presence of partner during birth, immediate contact with a healthy infant and absence of general anaesthesia were controlled. It is therefore not surprising that no significant differences were found in the psychological adjustment of these two groups of women as it is precisely the effects of general anaesthesia, lack of information, not having the partner present during the birth and separation from the baby immediately after birth that lead to many of the problems associated with caesarean delivery. It is interesting to note that even when these factors are controlled, a significant difference is still found between women who have been given a caesarean section and those who have delivered vaginally in terms of their satisfaction with their experience of childbirth. Such a difference could only be based on the mode of delivery.

Familiarity breeds content?

Some commentators have suggested that the increasing use of caesarean sections and the familiarity of the operation amongst expectant parents may itself contribute to new parents viewing the procedure as an alternative method of childbirth and therefore reduce any negative effects (Culp and Osofsky, 1989). It has even been proposed that as caesarean birth is so prevalent, women having the operation may feel 'normal' and not suffer in terms of distress or disappointment and that they may even feel 'special' (Shearer, 1989). However, there is no evidence available to support these claims.

SELF-HELP GROUPS

The growth in recent years of self-help groups for women who have had caesareans has been seen as indicating a clear psychological and social need for support which women who have undergone surgical delivery may feel, and some commentators have suggested that this represents a recognition among women of the effects that can follow from a caesarean section (Richards, 1983; Oakley and Richards, 1990). There is no doubting the value of such groups for women who need support and advice. It is also in this forum that women can explore perspectives other than those offered by the professionals and impose their own priorities and emphasis on to the subject matter. Trowell's 1986 study gave evidence to support the value of post-caesarean section support groups where mothers can feel free to discuss their own feelings and concerns about themselves.

However, the growth of such groups may indicate a cause for concern. First of all because it is unfortunate that support groups have become necessary. Perhaps if less caesareans were performed and women were better prepared for those operations that are necessary, there may be less need for support. Secondly, it is often the case that women from the lower socio-economic groups are excluded from support groups which are seen as 'middle class' enterprises. Women are excluded for many reasons including lack of information, access, time and experience. What this means is that many women who need support, help and advice will not get it. Surely it would be better to address women's needs prior to delivery rather than women having to organize themselves in order to provide the necessary support after the event.

Physiological effects

'Cesarean section is... the most important predisposing factor associated with maternal mortality and postpartum morbidity.' (Nielsen and Hökegárd, 1984, p. 106)

MORBIDITY

Caesarean birth is a major surgical procedure, and as such will always be associated with a morbidity rate greater than that of vaginal delivery. Serious maternal morbidity after the operation occurs in 9 to 15 per cent of caesarean sections (Engelkes and van Roosmalen, 1992). The major causes of post-operative morbidity being endometriosis, urinary tract infection and wound infection (NIH, 1981). The major abdominal surgery of caesarean section leaves many women tired with varying degrees of discomfort (Trowell, 1986) which may ultimately slow down the recovery process. In a North American study of recovery from childbirth, Tulman and Fawcett found that six months postpartum, 25 per cent of women did not feel physically recovered from the experience and caesarean section was found to be one of the major hindering factors to recovery (1991). British studies have also found that considerable maternal morbidity is associated with caesarean delivery (Francome et al., 1993) and that such effects can persist long after the birth (Hillan, 1992).

Women's experiences during delivery and the early postpartum can affect their perceptions of the birth. When childbirth is rated as painful and distressing, feelings about the experience are negative (Fawcett et al., 1992). One proposed solution to this problem is the increased use of analgesia in the early postpartum giving the mother more comfort and enabling her to bond with and care for her baby. Inadequate analgesia, it is suggested, leads to discomfort and insomnia which decreases the mother's ability to cope with all the physiological and psychological changes associated with the early postpartum (Macdonald, 1990).

Yet there is evidence to suggest that women's post-operative feelings of pain and physical distress can be decreased at the same time as enhancing their self-esteem, perceptions of the birth and feelings towards the baby by giving women appropriate information to enable them to come to terms with abdominal delivery (Wilson, 1981; Greene et al., 1989; Fawcett, 1990; Kanto et al., 1990). What this means is that post-operative morbidity can be decreased by greater preparation pre-operatively. This would reduce the need for increased analgesia post-operatively to enhance women's experience of caesarean section.

LONG TERM HEALTH EFFECTS

A Swedish study in 1991 comparing the long term health effects of women following caesarean section and vaginal deliveries found that whilst caesarean women had higher long term morbidity, as defined by use of hospital services, than those women who had a vaginal delivery, this morbidity was a continuation of previous (that is, prior to the caesarean operation) behaviour patterns for the women concerned. This suggests that poor health could be an indicator for caesarean section rather than a consequence of it. However the results did suggest an increase in problems during subsequent pregnancies, labours and deliveries for women who have had caesarean sections and that some of these problems may have been a consequence of the operation itself. More significantly, the study found an increased frequency of ectopic pregnancy following caesarean section (Hemminki, 1991). As many countries are now facing increasing rates of ectopic pregnancy, there is reason to suggest that further investigation is required into the relationship between caesarean section and subsequent ectopic pregnancies. Similarly, studies from Scotland and the United States found lower fertility rates among women following a caesarean section compared to women who had given birth vaginally (Hall et al., 1989), indicating that research into the effects of caesarean section on subsequent reproduction is imperative.

MATERNAL MORTALITY

Although the risk of death to mother and child from caesarean section may now be relatively small (compared to earlier times in the history of the operation), it is still a cause for concern as many deaths may be avoided. Caesarean section-related maternal mortality rates have decreased dramatically, in the United States, for example, the death rate from caesarean section declined from 0.11 per cent of all caesarean deliveries in 1970 to 0.04 per cent in 1978 (Guillemin, 1981). Yet deaths from caesarean birth still comprise the major part of total maternal mortality statistics. Similarly data from the UK shows that the numbers of deaths from caesareans have declined on the whole, even though the amount of caesareans being carried out have increased (Table 11.1).

Periods	Total deaths from caesareans	Total maternal deaths England and Wales	Total maternal deaths United Kingdom
1970–72	102 (E & W)		
1973–75	77 (E & W)	390	408
1976–78	80 (E & W)	325	
1979–81	87 (E & W)	268	
1982–84	69 (E & W)	209	
1985–87	64 (E & W)		
1988–90	85 (E & W)		
1985–87	76 (UK)		223
1988–90	91 (UK)		238

(Source: Department of Health, 1991 and 1994)

Table 11.1: Maternal deaths associated with caesarean section England and Wales 1970–90 and the United Kingdom 1985–90

Caesarean delivery is estimated to carry between two and eleven times the risk of maternal mortality compared to a vaginal delivery (Shearer, 1993) and caesareans performed because of previous caesareans carry twice the risk of maternal mortality of all vaginal deliveries (NIH, 1981). However, two early studies in the United States found the risk of death from caesarean section to be 10 to 26 times that for vaginal delivery (Evrad and Gold, 1977; Minkoff and Schwarcz, 1980). In England and Wales the estimated mortality from caesarean section was more than eight times greater than from vaginal delivery in 1972 (DHSS, 1975). In Sweden in the early 1980s the maternal mortality rate was 12.7 per 100,000 caesarean deliveries compared to 1.1 per 100,000 vaginal births, meaning that the risk of death from abdominal delivery was twelve times higher than that from vaginal birth (Moldin et al., 1984).

The latest data for the UK (published in 1994) concludes that there were 91 deaths following caesarean section for the three years 1988–90. The fall in mortality associated with caesareans observed in the previous triennium was not maintained. Care was judged to be substandard in relation to the management of the caesarean section and/ or after care in 21 of these cases (DoH, 1994).

Indications for caesarean section associated with maternal death in the UK (1988– 1990) were hypertensive disorders (n=15), antepartum haemorrhage (n=12), fetal distress (n=7), protracted labour (n=5) and previous caesarean section (n=3) (DoH, 1994).

The most common causes of death as a result of caesarean section are pulmonary embolism, hypertensive disorders and haemorrhage (DoH, 1994). Maternal deaths related to anaesthesia, although infrequent, continue to occur and most anaesthesia-related deaths are potentially avoidable. The frequency with which general anaesthesia is used for caesarean deliveries will inevitably influence the fatality rate. In England and Wales pulmonary embolism and complications of anaesthesia were identified as growing influences among specified causes of death associated with caesarean section in the 1970s. Deaths from these two causes have been classified as an 'inevitable risk of any pelvic operative procedure' (Chalmers and Richards, 1977, p. 43).

However, although there has been a substantial fall in deaths directly related to anaesthesia, it could be argued that if, as the literature suggests, many caesareans currently performed are unnecessary, the risk, however inevitable, is too much to ask any woman to take, particularly as the benefits to her about-to-be-born child are questionable.

Although it is not possible to compare changes in death rates from caesareans as a proportion of total maternal deaths, as maternal deaths will relate to total numbers of pregnancies and deliveries in any given year, the data presented in Table 11.1 is useful in demonstrating the fact that whilst maternal mortality rates overall have continued to decline, deaths from caesareans have not reduced substantially since the mid 1970s.[1] What this means is that maternal mortality rates may have reduced still further if caesarean section rates had not continued to rise.

---

1. The apparent increase in maternal deaths for 1988–90 compared to the previous triennium relates to an increase in the overall number of pregnancies over the period. The maternal mortality rate has not therefore changed.

The latest data available highlight a worrying trend whereby deaths associated with caesareans constitute a substantial proportion of the total maternal mortality in the United Kingdom, 34.1 per cent in 1985–1987 and 38.2 per cent in 1988 to 1990 (DoH, 1994). What this means is that if this trend continues, maternal mortality rates will be prevented from reaching their minimal level due to the continued use of caesarean section.

One of the most worrying issues arising from these data is that if, as the evidence suggests, many caesareans are carried out unnecessarily, many maternal deaths are potentially avoidable. In the United States it has been estimated that 140 women die each year following caesareans which were not medically indicated (Savage and Francome, 1993). Although the rate of caesarean sections performed in this country is only half that of the States, and therefore the number of maternal deaths associated with the operation correspondingly less, any level of maternal mortality is intolerable when operations are not necessary.

An increase in the rate of caesareans inevitably leads to an increase in the number of maternal deaths in childbirth. This has led some commentators to suggest that the increasing caesarean rates are responsible for the fact that maternal mortality rates have failed to decrease significantly during the last decades. The very serious implication here is that caesarean sections are responsible for keeping rates of maternal mortality relatively high. However, the reporting of maternal mortality is unsystematic and rates of maternal mortality are believed to be under-reported in a number of industrialized countries. The cause of death is often attributed to surgical procedures, such as anaesthesia accidents and thromboembolism, and are therefore recorded as deaths from surgery rather than deaths from childbirth. Similarly, the complex organization of many hospitals works against the accurate reporting of deaths that occur after transfer to intensive care units or after discharge and re-admission.

What is more, advances in anaesthetics and intensive care have also meant that the dividing line between mortality and severe morbidity has become less defined. Maternal mortality is therefore not necessarily a very reliable indicator of the effects of caesarean section. However, important differences do exist between countries, regions and hospitals (Derom et al., 1987) suggesting that differences in maternal mortality are more dependant on medical practice than differences in the populations of women served.

In Third World countries maternal mortality after caesarean section is much higher than in industrialized countries, as high as three per cent in some rural hospitals where general duty officers perform most operations, facilities for blood transfusion are scarce, anaesthetic practices poor and risks of infection high. This compares to a mortality rate of one per cent in teaching hospitals where conditions are better and more experienced staff are available (Engelkes and van Roosmalen, 1992). In Kaziba Hospital in rural Zaire where 12 per cent of births were by caesarean section in 1992, the risk of maternal mortality was 13 times higher for caesarean delivered women compared to vaginal deliveries. Many of the operations were performed by a nurse or dentist. Where the operations were carried out by those other than experienced doctors, a much higher rate of wound infection was observed (Onsrud and Onsrud, 1996). It appears therefore that deaths from caesarean section are influenced by the skills of the medical professionals, the availability of properly trained staff and adequate hospital services. Thus a high rate of caesarean section in countries with poorly developed health systems represents a greater risk to maternal health.

Caesarean section is, and will always be, a potentially dangerous operation for the mother, and the added hazard of anaesthesia, of whatever form, should not be underestimated. Although relatively small in number, there is a definite risk of death associated with the procedure. The more common the operation becomes, the more often women will die from causes associated with the procedure. The rates of maternal mortality related to caesarean section are still unacceptably high. For this reason it is imperative that the operation is only carried out in cases of real medical need and not for extraneous reasons, such as physicians' convenience, fear of litigation and financial considerations.

The effects of caesarean birth on the baby

The literature on the effects of caesarean birth on the baby is limited. The small number of studies conducted tend to concentrate on the first few months following the birth. Research on the long-term effects of caesarean birth on the child's development is, unfortunately, relatively scarce. The limited evidence available does not suggest that increases in the practice of caesarean deliveries has reduced infant morbidity and claims that reductions in perinatal mortality rates observed to coincide with increases in the caesarean section rate represent a causal relationship have not been proved (O'Driscoll and Foley, 1983; NIH, 1981). Cases of iatrogenic prematurity in caesarean births is at least one liability that has emerged from the common use of the procedure (Guillemin, 1981).

Physiological effects

The evidence suggests that respiratory distress in the newborn infant is higher after both primary caesarean (White et al., 1985) and repeat caesarean (NIH, 1981; Bowers et al., 1982) than after vaginal delivery. In a study assessing the excess risk to the infant delivered via repeat caesarean section independently of any risk associated with the indication for the procedure, Burt et al. concluded that some excess risk of low apgar scores may be associated with repeat caesarean section procedures (1988). Similarly the NIH report demonstrated that infants from both primary and repeat caesarean births had lower apgar scores than either forceps or spontaneous deliveries (1981). Further, it is not unrealistic to assume that babies will find caesarean birth more of a shock than spontaneous delivery, particularly when the operation is performed before the mother goes into labour. The incidence of respiratory distress syndrome is less amongst infants whose mothers are allowed to go into labour prior to the caesarean being performed than those whose mothers are operated on before the onset of labour (Cohen and Carson, 1985). This may indicate that the onset of labour is associated with greater preparedness for birth amongst infants. There is also evidence to suggest that this shock may make infants slower to breathe and have an effect on their ability to suck (Phillips, 1983).

Effects of anaesthesia and analgesics

Women who have caesareans are more likely to be given more anaesthesia and analgesic than those who deliver vaginally. The effect of these procedures on the baby are still a matter of controversy. The evidence available suggests that many analgesics and anaesthetics depress respiration in the newborn and may affect its ability to suck (Richards, 1983). Such effects may be of little consequence on there own, but coupled with other factors associated with abdominal delivery such as maternal depression, pain and immobility, these side-effects could become important stressors on the maternal/infant relationship.

Special/intensive care

It used to be routine practice in many hospitals to take the newborn baby to the Special Care Baby Unit (SCBU) following a caesarean delivery, regardless of the original reasons for the operation or the condition of the baby. During the 1970s, 20 per cent of all caesarean babies went to the SCBU for a time following their birth. Nearly half of these were perfectly healthy and not in need of specialist or intensive care (Phillips and Rakusen, 1978). Although the situation has improved, a proportion of caesarean babies are still routinely taken to the SCBU. The reasoning behind this appears to be that it is 'hospital policy' for certain types of delivery including caesarean and forceps. An alternative explanation could be that in times of strict management of resources it is simply more expedient to have a unit that is over-used in order to justify its existence. Whatever the rationale, it seems unnecessary to routinely admit caesarean babies to the SCBU unless there is a clear indication that specialist care or observation is necessary, particularly in the light of evidence suggesting a deleterious effect on bonding from early postpartum separation between mother and child (Klaus and Kennel, 1982).

Neonatal mortality

Both primary and repeat caesarean sections have consistently higher neonatal mortality rates than all vaginal births (NIH, 1981) and there is no evidence to suggest that higher caesarean section rates improve perinatal or neonatal outcomes.

Long term effects (psychological and developmental)

There is evidence to suggest that negative feelings towards the childbirth experience from the mother can have a long-term effect on the child, relating to problems in social-emotional adjustment. Brith et al. found that mothers who reported themselves to be anxious postpartum, those who thought it would be difficult to cope with the new situation at home and those who were assessed by the psychologist to be anxious or depressed, had children with more social-emotional difficulties at four years of age than mothers without these experiences (1992). Considering the evidence on the negative effects of caesarean section on the woman's experience of childbirth in terms of increased anxiety and depression it is not unreasonable to speculate that caesarean birth may have serious deleterious effects on the long-term development of the child.

However, it has been suggested that caesarean parents see their children in a more positive light than those experiencing vaginal delivery and that this leads to increased expectations from those children. An explanation offered for this is that caesarean-born children tend to have fewer siblings and, as a consequence, might receive more attention from their parents.[2]

Overall it appears that the benefits of caesarean section to babies in cases where abdominal delivery was not strictly necessary are dubious. Iatrogenic effects such as shock, difficulty in breathing and sucking, routine separation from the mother in the immediate postpartum period, together with increased risk of mortality indicate that a more selective approach to the use of caesarean section would be of benefit.

Effects of caesarean birth on the mother-child relationship

In view of the wealth of evidence pointing to negative side-effects of caesarean section for both the mother and her child, it is not unreasonable to assume that these responses will have some repercussions on the mother-child relationship.

The different perceptions of caesarean mothers about their birth experiences, and subsequently their children, compared to women who deliver vaginally may have an effect on the children of caesarean births. Whilst no objective differences in the children born by caesarean and those born vaginally are evident as yet, caesarean mothers have been found to perceive their children to be more difficult, tend to find discipline a problem and have less complete immunization schedules for their children. They feel that their babies develop into a person later, have less eye-to-eye contact and rate their infants less optimally on revised infant temperament questionnaires (Trowell, 1989; Simons et al., 1992). However, overall physical contact has not been found to be different (Trowell, 1989). Such evidence would suggest that the effects of the birth experience does have a lasting, and possibly detrimental, effect on the relationship between mother and child.

Bonding

For bonding to occur appropriately it is necessary for early mother-infant contact to take place, especially during the first hour after delivery (Klaus and Kennel, 1982). Similarly, it appears that early and extended contact between mother and child can greatly influence a mother's interaction with her child, their relationship, and ultimately the child's development (Kennel et al., 1974). This has serious implications for women who have their babies by caesarean as many are separated from their newborns immediately after birth. Frequently caesarean infants spend 24 hours or more under observation in special care units often due to hospital routine or policy rather than

---

2. The number of siblings of caesarean-born children may be fewer because women with caesarean births are often advised to limit their childbearing (Entwisle and Alexander, 1987). Furthermore, some women may decide not to have any more children because of negative perceptions about childbirth as a result of caesarean section (Hillan, 1992).

medical need (NIH, 1981; Huntingford, 1985). Hillan found that amongst her study group of women delivering by caesarean section, almost half did not hold their babies in the 12 hours following the birth and 76 per cent did not feed their babies in the 24 hours after delivery. Amongst the control group of women who had delivered vaginally, 90 per cent held their babies immediately after birth and 92 per cent fed their babies within 24 hours of birth (1992). This early separation of mother and child following caesarean birth can have a significant impact on their subsequent relationship.

What is more, when women have had caesareans, it is often the case that when the first contact does occur, it comes at a time when the mother is in pain and/or when she is drowsy from the effects of anaesthesia and medication. Not surprisingly women delivered by caesarean section take significantly longer to feel close to their babies than those delivered vaginally (Hillan, 1992). A study comparing the mother-infant relationship during the first postpartum visit of caesarean-delivered women and those delivered vaginally showed a difference between the two groups in the frequency and amount of handling of the infants in that the caesarean mothers handled their babies significantly less (Tulman, 1986). The difference in maternal attitude and behaviour towards the child appears to be related to caesarean birth rather than intervention in the birth process per se as no statistical difference was found amongst women having vaginal deliveries between those women delivered by forceps and those delivering spontaneously (Hillan, 1992).

Therefore it appears that close contact between the mother and her infant post-caesarean section could improve their relationship and aid the bonding process. However, current post-caesarean practice in many hospitals is denying women this opportunity.

Long-term effects

Evidence suggests that caesarean birth may have a deleterious effect on the mother's relationship with her child over a long period of time. Studies have shown that early contact between the mother and her newborn is important, not only for bonding but for the mother-child relationship throughout the early years of the child's life. For example, a study by Marut and Mercer comparing the experiences of women who had had caesarean sections under general anaesthetic with those of women who had had unproblematic vaginal deliveries found that the caesarean mothers' comments about their infants reflected hostility, whereas the vaginal delivery mothers' remarks reflected concern (1979). This implies that mothers who are denied close physical contact with their newborns, as many caesarean patients are, particularly those having emergency operations under general anaesthetic, are also being denied the opportunity to develop a close and loving bond with their babies at the crucial time.

Trowell, in her work comparing the mother-child relationship between a study group of women who had had emergency caesareans and a control group of women who had delivered vaginally, found that one month after the birth the emergency caesarean group mothers had less eye-to-eye contact with their babies than the control group and were less relaxed when bathing their babies. Further, the majority of the study group recollected the birth as a bad experience and expressed concern about their own ability to care for their babies. One year after the birth the study group expressed more dissatisfaction and resentment at the demands made on them by their babies and felt that they had experienced more problems during the first year. They also responded more slowly to their child crying (1983).

The findings of these studies have major implications for the use of caesarean section concerning the long-term effects of operative birth. Some commentators have gone further and raised alarm regarding the over-use of caesarean section with the accompanying separation of mother and child in the immediate postpartum. Perhaps the most worrying long-term effect of caesarean section that has been suggested by two studies is child abuse. Both Lynch and Roberts (1977) and Caffo et al. (1982) identified caesarean delivery as a factor associated with later child abuse.[3]

> 'The disproportionately high percentage of mothering disturbances, such as child abuse and deprivation, failure to thrive, which occur after a mother has been separated from her... newborn infant, force a thorough review and evaluation of our present perinatal practices.' (Kennel et al., 1974)

It is clear that further research into the long term effects of caesarean birth on the mother-child relationship is essential.

Breastfeeding

The evidence available on the relationship between caesarean section and breastfeeding is inconclusive. Studies from around the world have suggested that caesarean delivered women are less likely to breastfeed than those who deliver vaginally (Marut and Mercer, 1979; Goteborgs, 1987; Janke, 1988; Forman et al., 1991; Mathur et al, 1993; Ever-Hadani et al., 1994). This appears to be the case, particularly for women who have operations under general, rather than regional, anaesthetic. Women who have regional anaesthesia for their caesareans tend to feel less tired, depressed and more mobile thereby enabling them to begin breastfeeding sooner than those women who have received general anaesthesia. The difficulties appear to persist so that even when breastfeeding is successfully established, less caesarean-delivered women continue to breastfeed compared to those who deliver spontaneously (Menghetti et al., 1994).

In contrast, an earlier study of breastfeeding outcomes to determine the impact of caesarean delivery found that although mothers giving birth by caesarean had a later first breastfeeding than those who delivered vaginally, there was no relationship between delivery type and duration of breastfeeding or pain or fatigue related to breastfeeding duration (Kearney et al., 1990). It appears that a high level of commitment to breastfeeding from the mothers is associated with breastfeeding success irrespective of birth type (Janke, 1988; Kearney et al., 1990). However, caesarean section does affect women's ease and comfort in breastfeeding as the incision makes feeding more difficult in that finding a comfortable position for holding the baby presents a major problem (Sargent and Stark, 1987; Francome et al., 1993).

---

3. Neither of these studies reported the statistical significance of their results and as such should be interpreted with caution.

Overall, the evidence once again points to a more conservative use of caesarean section coupled with a review of routine procedures of dubious value to the health of mother and child such as early postpartum separation.

In conclusion, it appears that the negative effects of caesarean birth on women are related to: use of general anaesthesia, absence of a partner or friend during delivery, lack of detailed information about the events surrounding caesarean birth, missing out on vaginal delivery, having a longer recovery time, experiencing greater pain, routine separation of the infant from the mother at birth as is common practice, emergency rather than elective operations and most importantly, the increased risk of fatality from childbirth.

For the babies of caesareans the evidence does not point to better outcomes physiologically or psychologically and caesarean birth actually increases iatrogenic risks, including higher rates of infant mortality. Furthermore, it has been suggested that caesarean birth affects the long term relationship between the mother and child for reasons associated with surgical delivery alone.

The sheer volume of evidence pointing to the negative effects of caesarean section highlight the very real need for obstetricians to take a good look at their own practices and ensure that every caesarean is a necessary operation. Where abdominal birth is considered to be the best option available, women should be given regional rather than general anaesthesia, be allowed to have a companion with them and not be separated from their babies immediately after delivery unless this is absolutely necessary. Furthermore, women should be made fully aware of all the risks, so that they know what to expect, and can make informed decisions wherever possible.

Reducing the negative effects of caesarean birth

The evidence suggests that giving information to expectant parents prior to delivery can enhance reactions to unplanned caesarean birth in terms of decreasing the amount of pain and physical distress experienced whilst increasing self-esteem, enhancing feelings towards the baby and making perceptions of the birth experience more positive (Fawcett and Burritt, 1985; Fawcett, 1990). This looks likely to be the case as previous studies found that pre-operative information given during a personal visit from an anaesthetist was linked with patients feeling less pain post-operatively, requiring fewer analgesics, making a speedier recovery from the anaesthetic and having a shorter stay in hospital (Egbert et al., 1964; Wilson, 1981). Similarly, it appears that a pre-operative visit by an anaesthetic nurse to give information about surgery and anaesthetic has benefits for patients post-operatively in terms of reduced anxiety and related symptoms including reduced use of analgesics and earlier ambulation (Kanto et al., 1990). Further, an evaluation of the effects of sensory information about caesarean delivery on prenatal maternal anxiety and on subsequent recovery found that the patients who were given the information showed less physiologenic arousal during surgery and enhanced postsurgical recovery (Greene et al., 1989).

It appears that information about caesarean birth given to women pre-operatively enhances their post-operative experience both physically and psychologically. Being better informed about caesarean section helps women adjust emotionally to operative delivery and reduces the likelihood of women suffering long-term psychological disturbance as a result of thwarted expectations (Nolan, 1990).

Negative reactions to childbirth amongst caesarean patients detailed in this chapter suggest that women need to be more adequately prepared at the antenatal stage and that the possibility of having a caesarean birth needs to be impressed upon all pregnant women in order that they may acquire the information and knowledge that they will need in the event of a caesarean being deemed necessary. Many authors have stressed this point and suggested that information on caesarean delivery should be given to all women irrespective of whether they are thought to be 'at risk' or not. This recommendation is not new, childbirth educators had begun to take account of this necessity during the 1970s (Conklin, 1977; Conner, 1977; Enkin, 1977) and in 1981 the National Institutes of Health Consensus Task Force stressed the point in the United States.

Women have also been shown to equate advance information, whether in the form of an antenatal class, reading material, or as a cautionary statement from a physician, with a state of preparedness (Sargent and Stark, 1987). When asked specifically which type of information they require, women's suggestions have included: issues surrounding caesarean birth, advantages and disadvantages of different types of anaesthesia, reasons for and effects of different surgical incisions, more emphasis on emotional reactions to caesarean birth, and details about the medical and surgical complications associated with caesarean delivery (Fawcett and Burritt, 1985; Francome et al., 1993; see also pp. 126–127).

However, results of studies on the effect of information about caesarean birth given to expectant parents are not conclusive and some researchers have found that childbirth classes influence responses to delivery less than pre-existing beliefs, values and expectations (Sargent and Stark, 1989; Beal, 1993). Others have found no significant differences between women given comprehensive caesarean birth information and those given standard childbirth information in terms of their perceptions of the birth experience, physical distress, self-esteem, functional status, feelings about the baby, or quality of the marital relationship (Fawcett et al., 1993). However, the majority of research in this area has been carried out in the United States and it has been suggested that the current high caesarean section rate may itself encourage expectant and new parents to view caesarean birth as a normal or alternative mode of delivery (Culp and Osofsky, 1989).

It has been argued that as childbirth classes now routinely address the possibility of caesarean birth and attempt to prepare expectant parents for a surgical delivery, the negative sentiments following abdominal delivery may become less prevalent, mitigated by preparation (Sargent and Stark, 1987). It is certainly the case that many pregnant women do attend antenatal classes. Hillan found that 76 per cent of her sample of women had attended at least one antenatal class (1992). The results of studies on the effects of antenatal education, including information on caesarean birth, continue to suggest that expectant parents need to be prepared for unanticipated caesarean delivery (Fawcett and Henklein, 1987). However this is not occurring from current antenatal education practice, despite the inclusion of information on caesarean section. Comments made by childbirth educators consistently indicate that content about caesarean delivery routinely presented in childbirth classes does not prepare expectant parents for the possibility of caesarean delivery (Fawcett and Burritt, 1985). It appears that expectant parents are reluctant to accept the information regarding surgical delivery or even attend the classes relating specifically to it, probably because they see it as something that happens to other people, particularly when their own pregnancy has been unproblematic. One respondent in a study designed to investigate the value of information on caesarean birth in the form of a detailed pamphlet to expectant parents still reported that he 'thought it wouldn't happen to us' (Fawcett and Burritt, 1985, p. 227).

Thus it appears that there continues to be a lack of realistic preparation for the possibility of surgical birth among women having babies. It has been suggested that expectant parents not only need information on caesarean birth in the form of antenatal class or printed material, but that the message needs to be emphasized by a follow-up home visit or telephone call to reinforce the information (Fawcett and Burritt, 1985). In their study Fawcett and Burritt found such arrangements to be beneficial to expectant parents in that it provided an opportunity for clarification of the written material and provision of additional information about pregnancy in general and caesarean birth in particular.

Further, it appears that giving information to women about caesarean birth prior to delivery not only enhances their childbirth experience but may actually have an effect on intervention rates. This is because better-informed patients may question levels of intervention and be in a position to discuss the relative benefits and hazards of the available procedures. It is more likely, however, to do with the fact that practitioners who deem it important to keep women informed at all stages of delivery are also the ones more likely to be questioning their own practices in the light of evidence suggesting that increased levels of intervention do not necessarily improve maternal and perinatal outcomes. A study in Vienna found that a pre-childbirth educational programme of intensive preparation together with a policy of minimal intervention in delivery reduced the incidence of caesarean section to 1.3 per cent (Rockenschaub, 1990).

CHAPTER TWELVE

Women's Experience of Caesarean Birth

Part I: The Research

This research consists of two studies on women's experiences of caesarean section: a major research project conducted in 1991/2 and a follow-up survey in 1996.

With the current emphasis on 'consumer choice' in health care services, it is a matter of concern that there are virtually no public disclosure requirements placed on practitioners that would make them provide information to their customers (patients) about the quality of their services or their competence to perform these services. Therefore when doctors recommend a particular course of action or type of treatment to pregnant women, they do not have to support their recommendations with evidence. It appears that the popular tenet 'doctor knows best' overrides the need to justify medical decisions. What is more worrying is that when women are advised about the appropriate course of action, they may not be given the information they need to make informed decisions. As evidence presented in Chapter 8 demonstrates, at best women are misinformed, at worst they are lied to. What this means is that women make decisions (or agree to decisions) that may not be in their best interest. Caesarean sections provide a powerful and contemporary example of how women are often steered towards one course of treatment when another less invasive one may be appropriate.

Theory of research

Previous research on caesarean section has exhaustively analyzed the indications for the operation, reasons for the increasing rate and women's perceptions of childbirth in general and surgical delivery in particular. This study differs, in eliciting responses from women on a range of issues relating to caesarean birth and by comparing the information given to women over a five year period. Although much research has been carried out on being better informed about caesarean birth and the effect it has on the outcome of the operation for the women involved, what is missing from the current literature is an examination of how women who have caesareans in hospitals in Britain feel about the amount of information offered to them, their treatment and the effect of caesarean birth in general.

The theory underpinning this research is that if women are to be offered the best possible maternity care, what they need is to be assured that every caesarean is necessary and, when necessary, that women are properly and fully informed of all that is happening and what the after-effects are likely to be. If women are to make informed choices about how they want to deliver their babies, what support and help they will need and what medical treatment, if any, is suitable, they need from health care professionals accurate, consistent information imparted at a level that women can understand, from a professional that they have been able to establish a relationship with and whom they trust. Only then will women be empowered to have control over what happens to them in hospital and be able to have a sense of achievement through having participated in the decision-making process leading to feelings of greater satisfaction with the experience of childbirth.

The increased use of interventionist techniques in childbirth have not led to improvements in perinatal morbidity or mortality and could be responsible for increases in iatrogenic effects, as well as higher maternal morbidity and possible long term deleterious effects on the mother-child relationship. It is my contention, therefore, that less use of interventionist techniques, caesarean section in particular, coupled with appropriately informed expectant women, will lead to a better outcome for the mother, child and health care professional.

Hypotheses and research questions

Evidence suggests that more caesareans are being performed than can be justified in terms of neonatal/perinatal or maternal outcomes. Too many caesareans are performed for extraneous reasons, such as fear of litigation, rather than medical necessity. The evidence available suggests that caesarean birth has a detrimental effect on women. The aim of the research was to investigate women's experiences of caesarean section.

Hypothesis One: Caesarean birth denies women the opportunity to have a satisfying experience of childbirth and increases their suffering.

Research question One: Do women suffer as a result of caesarean sections?

Hypothesis Two: Maternity services can be improved with regard to caesarean section to ensure a better outcome for women.

Research question Two: What can be done to improve the outcome for women of childbirth in general, and caesarean section in particular?

Methods

This research utilized a survey design, together with interviews, to assess the experiences of women having caesarean sections. The aim of the survey was, first, to find out from women the reasons they had been given for their operations and to provide an overall picture of the pattern of caesarean birth in England, Scotland and Wales. Secondly, to analyze women's experiences of caesarean birth in the light of current debate on the effects of medical intervention and suggest ways in which the management of birth can best be achieved to ensure a satisfactory outcome for all concerned.

The latter study was based on the same survey design and conducted to provide data on changes in women's experiences over the five year period 1991/2 to 1996.

The sampling procedure

In 1991/2 a sample consisting of one hospital from each of the Health Authority regions was randomly selected to represent the region. Permission to conduct the survey of women's experiences was requested from Consultant Obstetricians responsible in each case. Eleven hospitals, geographically spread across the country, agreed to participate in the study, the remainder either failed to respond or declined to take part. The two-page questionnaires were sent out along with covering letters to the participating hospitals with the request that they be handed to 50 consecutive women who had had caesareans and who agreed to complete the questionnaire.

In order to maximize comparability of sample population between 1991/2 and 1996 the eight hospitals who returned completed questionnaires in the 1991/2 study were contacted and asked to participate in the follow-up survey. All agreed.

The questionnaire

The 1991/2 questionnaire asked for quantitative data about the women, the operations and the babies, as well as qualitative information regarding the women's experiences and feelings about the births. The questionnaires were coded and entered on to a computer where the data were analyzed. The questionnaire was amended slightly for the follow-up study on the basis of issues identified in the earlier study (see Appendices I and II for examples of the covering letter to participants and questionnaire).

THE RESPONSE RATE

In 1991/2 three hundred completed questionnaires were received from eight of the 11 hospitals that agreed to participate, that is, a response rate of 73 per cent. The number of questionnaires received from each hospital varied from 20 to 50. In 1996 the eight participating hospitals returned completed questionnaires by the cut-off date.

Fifty questionnaires were received from four hospitals. One hospital did not take responsibility for collecting questionnaires (at their request) and so return envelopes were distributed with the forms. This resulted in a response rate of 30 from 50 questionnaires distributed. The remaining four hospitals were requested to discontinue distribution and submit completed questionnaires for analysis resulting in 18 questionnaires from one hospital reporting that their caesarean section rate had been very low of late. Another sent 33. One hospital had been unable to commence with questionnaire distribution until quite late in the research programme due to the amount of audit at local, regional and national level. However, they were able to supply 27 completed questionnaires by the cut-off date. This resulted in a total sample of 308 questionnaires.

The interviews

Formal and informal interviews were conducted with seventeen women who had caesareans. Interviewees volunteered by indicating that they would like to participate further in the study at the end of the questionnaire they had completed in hospital. Therefore interviewees were already part of the survey sample and their data included as such. The purpose of the interviews was to support the findings of the survey and add to the qualitative evidence in the results.

Formal interviews were semi-structured based on the survey questionnaire. Women were given the opportunity to expand on answers given in the questionnaire and add any information they deemed relevant.

The sample

Information on parity, age and type of caesarean (elective or emergency) show that the demographic features of the sample population have remained stable over the five year period of study.

Of the three hundred caesareans in the 1991/2 sample 132 (44.0 per cent) were elective and 168 (56.0 per cent) were emergency operations. The 1996 sample constituted 143 (46.4 per cent) elective and 165 (53.6 per cent) emergency caesareans.

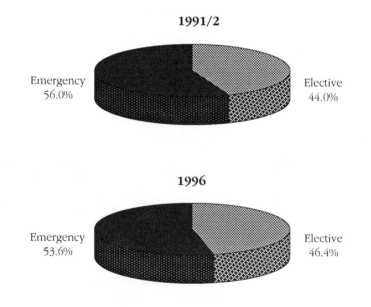

Fig. 12.1: Elective and emergency caesareans, 1991/2 and 1996

The respondents were further divided into three categories: primigravidae, previous vaginal deliveries and previous deliveries including caesareans. The data were tabulated as follows:

YEAR	Elective				Emergency				All caesareans			
	1991/2		**1996**		1991/2		**1996**		1991/2		**1996**	
	n	%	***n***	**%**	*n*	%	***n***	**%**	*n*	%	***n***	**%**
Primigravidae	27	20.5	**36**	**25.2**	115	68.5	**113**	**68.5**	142	47.3	**149**	**48.4**
Previous vaginal deliveries	25	18.9	**41**	**28.7**	36	21.4	**44**	**26.7**	61	20.4	**85**	**27.6**
Previous caesarean sections	80	60.6	**66**	**46.1**	17	10.1	**8**	**4.8**	97	32.3	**74**	**24.0**
Total	132	100	**143**	**100**	168	100	**165**	**100**	300	100	**308**	**100**

Table 12.1: Elective and emergency caesareans by previous birth history, 1991/2 and 1996

Overall numbers of primigravidae in the study have remained constant over the five year period of study. Almost half the operations were carried out on women giving birth for the first time. Some reduction in the number of repeat caesareans is evident. However, there has been a slight increase in caesareans for women with previous vaginal deliveries particularly in the elective category.

Age

Respondents were divided into seven age bands. The data were tabulated as follows:

AGE	Elective				Emergency				All caesareans			
	1991/2		**1996**		1991/2		**1996**		1991/2		**1996**	
	n	%	***n***	**%**	*n*	%	***n***	**%**	*n*	%	***n***	**%**
15–19	6	4.6	**4**	**2.8**	11	6.6	**14**	**8.5**	17	5.8	**18**	**5.9**
20–24	14	10.9	**22**	**15.4**	35	21.1	**24**	**14.5**	49	16.6	**46**	**14.9**
25–29	43	33.3	**43**	**30.0**	55	33.1	**58**	**35.2**	98	33.2	**101**	**32.8**
30–34	45	34.9	**48**	**33.6**	48	28.9	**47**	**28.5**	93	31.5	**95**	**30.9**
35–39	18	14.0	**22**	**15.4**	16	9.7	**16**	**9.7**	34	11.5	**38**	**12.3**
40–44	2	1.5	**3**	**2.1**	1	0.6	**5**	**3.0**	3	1.0	**8**	**2.6**
45+	1	0.8	**1**	**0.7**	0	0.0	**1**	**0.6**	1	0.4	**2**	**0.6**
Total	129	100	**143**	**100**	166	100	**165**	**100**	295	100	**308**	**100**

Women who did not answer are excluded from this table

Table 12.2: Age of women having caesareans, 1991/2 and 1996

The age at which women have caesareans has remained constant over the five year period of study. Some change is evident in the lower age groups (<24) where the 1996 data shows little difference between emergency and elective operations yet the earlier study demonstrated higher numbers of emergency operations in women under 24 years of age. As would be expected from the childbearing population the majority of women having caesareans were aged between 20 and 39 years. Almost two in three were between 25 and 34 years old (see Figure 12.2).

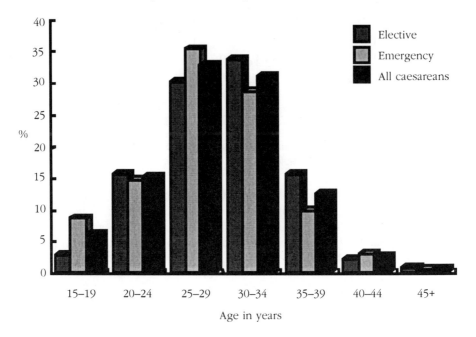

Fig. 12.2: Age of women having caesareans, 1996

In 1991/2 the four women in the sample who were over 40 years of age had elective caesareans, all had previously given birth including at least one previous caesarean. However, the reasons for these caesareans were not to do with their age but other conditions such as previous caesareans, breech presentation and cephalopelvic disproportion. In the latest study there were ten women over 40, four elective and six emergency operations. The elective operations were performed for previous caesarean, oblique presentation, high blood pressure, large baby anticipated, previous problems following vaginal forceps delivery and in two cases due to maternal age. Indications for emergency operations among women over 40 in the sample were previous caesarean, baby small for dates, cephalopelvic disproportion, dystocia in four cases, high blood pressure in two cases and maternal age in two cases. Thus age was mentioned as an indicator for caesareans in only four cases of women over 40 years of age. Interestingly four women in the 35 to 39 age group cited age as a reason for their operations, three were 38, one was 35.

Stage of pregnancy when caesareans performed

Women were asked 'How many weeks pregnant were you when your baby was born?'.

NO. OF WEEKS	Elective				Emergency				All caesareans			
	1991/2		1996		1991/2		1996		1991/2		1996	
	n	%	*n*	%	*n*	%	*n*	%	*n*	%	*n*	%
30	0	0.0	0	0.0	3	1.8	0	0.0	3	1.0	0	0.0
31	0	0.0	2	1.4	1	0.6	1	0.6	1	0.3	3	1.0
32	1	0.8	0	0.0	3	1.8	2	1.2	4	1.3	2	0.6
33	2	1.5	1	0.7	0	0.0	3	1.8	2	0.7	4	1.3
34	1	0.8	1	0.7	5	3.0	6	3.6	6	2.0	7	2.3
35	1	0.8	3	2.1	4	2.4	5	3.0	5	1.7	8	2.6
36	6	4.5	4	2.8	6	3.6	7	4.2	12	4.0	11	3.6
37	11	8.3	16	11.2	11	6.5	10	6.0	22	7.3	26	8.4
38	55	41.7	75	52.4	16	9.5	14	8.5	71	23.7	89	28.9
39	27	20.4	29	20.3	22	13.1	26	15.8	49	16.3	55	17.9
40	22	16.7	3	2.1	40	23.8	40	24.4	62	20.7	43	13.9
41	2	1.5	4	2.8	38	22.6	35	21.2	40	13.3	39	12.7
42	1	0.8	1	0.7	15	8.9	15	9.1	16	5.3	16	5.2
43	0	0.0	0	0.0	0	0.0	1	0.6	0	0.0	1	0.3
N/A	3	2.2	4	2.8	4	2.4	0	0.0	7	2.4	4	1.3
Total	132	100	143	100	168	100	165	100	300	100	308	100

Table 12.3: Number of weeks pregnant when caesareans performed, 1991/2 and 1996

Data from the two studies demonstrate a concentration of caesarean operations between weeks 38 and 41 of pregnancy when almost three quarters of operations were performed. However, differences emerge when comparing the caesareans that were done as an emergency and those that were elective (see Figure 12.3). Over a half (52.4 per cent) elective caesareans were carried out at week 38 whereas only one in twelve (8.5 per cent) emergency caesareans were done at this time. The largest proportion of emergency caesareans were performed on or after week 39 with three in five (61.4 per cent) being carried out between weeks 39 and 41.

The results therefore show that, on average, emergency caesareans are performed later in pregnancy than elective caesareans, presumably because such operations are often performed after a trial of labour. However, with elective caesareans there is no necessity to wait for the woman to go into labour and the decision about when to operate is left to the doctors. Caesarean surgery is usually arranged for the 39th week of pregnancy. The results are therefore consistent with accepted practice regarding the timing of elective caesarean operations.

There appears to be an 'optimum' or 'preferred' time for performing caesareans at around 38 weeks. Such decisions are based on the belief that there is an ideal gestation period and that the majority of women will fall into this statistical category. However, such notions could be problematic for women who do not, as these women are still likely to be given caesarean sections at this time. This may have serious implications

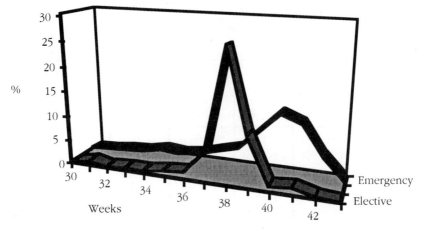

Fig. 12.3: Number of weeks pregnant when caesareans performed, 1996

for the babies of women who have longer than average gestation periods in that it means that they may be delivered too early. Similarly, for women whose natural gestation is less than average, their babies will be left in-utero too long and this could have a deleterious effect on both mother and child. Decisions on when to operate are made on the basis of a combination of factors which take into consideration the size and condition of the baby as well as the physical and mental state of the woman.

The babies

WEIGHT OF BABIES AT BIRTH

Mothers were asked: 'How much did your baby weigh at birth?'. The results were:

WEIGHT IN KILOGRAMS	Elective				Emergency				All caesareans			
	1991/2		**1996**		1991/2		**1996**		1991/2		**1996**	
	n	%	**n**	**%**	n	%	**n**	**%**	n	%	**n**	**%**
1,000–1,499	0	0.0	**0**	**0.0**	2	1.2	**1**	**0.7**	2	0.7	**1**	**0.4**
1,500–1,999	1	0.8	**3**	**2.3**	5	3.1	**5**	**3.4**	6	2.2	**8**	**2.9**
2,000–2,499	4	3.3	**6**	**4.6**	12	7.6	**11**	**7.4**	16	5.7	**17**	**6.1**
2,500–2,999	31	25.2	**25**	**19.4**	23	14.6	**19**	**12.8**	54	19.2	**44**	**15.9**
3,000–3,499	36	29.3	**46**	**35.6**	50	31.6	**31**	**20.9**	86	30.7	**77**	**27.8**
3,500–3,999	36	29.3	**40**	**31.0**	38	24.1	**55**	**37.2**	74	26.3	**95**	**34.3**
4,000–4,499	11	8.9	**5**	**3.9**	20	12.7	**22**	**14.9**	31	11.0	**27**	**9.7**
4,500–4,999	3	2.4	**2**	**1.6**	8	5.1	**4**	**2.7**	11	3.9	**6**	**2.2**
5,000–5,499	1	0.8	**0**	**0.0**	0	0.0	**0**	**0.0**	1	0.3	**0**	**0.0**
5,500–6,000	0	0.0	**2**	**1.6**	0	0.0	**0**	**0.0**	0	0.0	**2**	**0.7**
Total	123	100	**129**	**100**	158	100	**148**	**100**	281	100	**277**	**100**

Women who did not answer and twin births are excluded from this table

Table 12.4: Caesarean babies' weight at birth (singletons), 1991/2 and 1996

The results reveal that almost four in five (78.0 per cent) caesarean babies were delivered at the 2,500 kilograms (kg) to 3,999 kg weight range. The overall population of caesarean babies in the two studies are the same. A slight shift in the mode weight of babies is evident between 1991/2 and 1996. In the 1991/2 survey more babies were born at 3,000 to 3,499 kg whereas the 1996 data show the 3,500 to 3,999 kg weight range to have the highest number.

The birth weight of babies from emergency operations tended to span the weight range more than those from elective operations. They also peak at a higher weight than babies from elective operations which showed a definite peak at 3,000 kg to 3,499 kg in 1996 (see Figure 12.4). These data indicate that elective caesareans are increasingly carried out at what is perceived by the medical practitioners to be the 'ideal' size and decisions are based very much upon calculations of 'average' babies. As with calculations of average gestation periods, average size and weight of babies may have important implications for babies who, for a number of reasons, do not fall within the average.

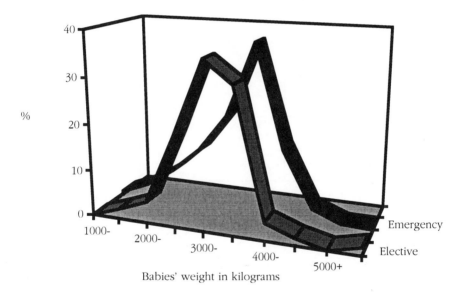

Fig. 12.4: Weight of caesarean babies at birth, 1996

Results

The operation

REASONS FOR CAESAREAN SECTION

The mothers were asked: 'What reason(s) did the doctors give for performing a caesarean operation?. You may have been given more than one reason so please tick the answers that apply to you'. There followed a list of 'reasons' and space for women to add any reasons given to them that were not included in the list. The results were tabulated as follows:

	1991/2		1996	
	n	%	*n*	%
repeat caesarean	87	29.0	74	24.0
dystocia	74	24.7	67	21.7
fetal distress	62	20.7	61	19.8
cephalopelvic disproportion	86	28.7	60	19.5
breech presentation	57	19.0	53	17.2
baby was small for dates	7	2.3	15	4.9
transverse lie	9	3.0	14	4.5
high blood pressure	7	2.3	13	4.2
antepartum haemorrhage	16	5.3	10	3.2
cord around baby's neck	13	4.3	10	3.2
diabetes	6	2.0	10	3.2
maternal age	5	1.7	8	2.6
twins	2	0.7	7	2.3
placenta praevia	3	1.0	4	1.3
cord prolapse	3	1.0	2	0.6
Other reasons	48	16.0	42	13.6
Total no. reasons	485		450	
Average no. reasons per woman	1.6		1.5	
Total no. women	300		308	

Percentages total more than 100 as many women were given a number of reasons for their caesareans

Table 12.5: Reasons for caesarean sections, 1991/2 and 1996

Reasons for caesarean section have remained constant over the five year period of study. The results show that some women were given as many as three or four reasons for caesarean section and others only one. On average 1.5 reasons were given per woman. The latest data show that the reasons given to women were quite widespread. For example, almost a quarter (24.0 per cent) of the sample were told that their caesareans were necessary because they had previous caesareans. A slightly smaller number (21.7 per cent) were told that labour was taking a long time (dystocia). Almost one in five (19.8 per cent) were told that their babies were distressed and a similar number (19.5 per cent) were told that their babies were too big for their pelves. Just over one in six (17.2 per cent) were given caesareans because their babies were in breech position. Explanations given in the 'Other reasons' section showed no commonalities between caesareans performed as emergencies and operations performed electively.

Reasons given to women for their caesareans vary. However they can be ranked as follows, beginning with the most common reason:

1. Repeat caesareans (24.0 per cent in 1996, 29.0 per cent in 1991/2)

Almost a quarter of women were told that their caesareans were necessary because they had previous caesareans. From the data obtained in this study it is not possible to say whether this was because of hospital policy of 'once a caesarean, always a caesarean'. However, a survey of consultants' attitudes towards caesarean section revealed that less than one in fifty consultants in England and Wales adheres to this policy (Francome et al., 1993) and so it is unlikely that it is this dictum which is responsible for the high number of repeat caesareans. It is therefore more likely that repeat caesareans are one of the most common indicators for the operation because the reasons for the previous operation, for example, size of pelvis, will remain the same. It may also be that women request elective operations because of their previous experiences of trial of labour which ended in caesarean section. If this is the case, it reflects lack of information given to women about the feasibility and value of VBAC.

2. Dystocia (21.7 per cent in 1996, 24.7 per cent in 1991/2)

One in five women were told that their caesareans were necessary because their labour was taking a long time. Although this reason may accompany other reasons such as fetal distress, it is still a surprisingly high proportion. One in five women in the study were not able to deliver within what are perceived to be the appropriate timescales and therefore subjected to operative delivery. Yet medical estimates of what constitutes a long labour vary. In the British Birth Survey of 1958, twenty four hours was considered long (Butler and Bonham, 1963). By 1970, eighteen hours was taken as the time beyond which a labour was deemed long (Chamberlain and Chamberlain, 1975). A British survey in the early 1990s found that of 39 consultants who said that they put a time limit on labour, just over half (20) said the limit was twelve hours. One consultant said he considered the labour long and the woman in need of a caesarean 'if the sun had set twice on her labour'. The longest time limit for labour given by one consultant was thirty six hours (Francome et al., 1993, p. 67).

It has been suggested that intervention in childbirth is accelerated by an emphasis on time scales combined with a rigid adherence to the three stages of labour (Savage, 1986). The results of the present study certainly add weight to this argument. This raises concerns over who decides what are the appropriate timescales and on what basis such decisions are made. However, when comparing the results of this study with those of the survey of consultant's attitudes to caesarean section, an interesting difference emerges. Almost nine out of ten (89.4 per cent) consultants in England and Wales said that they placed no time limit on labour when deciding to perform a caesarean (Francome et al., 1993), yet one in five women in the current study were told that their labour was taking too long.

This discrepancy can be explained in two ways. The first explanation is that women are not being told the truth about the reasons for their caesareans. It does not necessarily mean that women are being deliberately lied to, but rather that, for a variety of reasons, women are not being given the full explanation. This may be because doctors do not want to upset women, particularly in a situation where they may already be distressed because of a long and painful labour. Women are therefore told that they are having a caesarean because the labour is taking too long rather than being told that the baby is in distress or that there may be something more seriously wrong with the baby. Similarly, women may not be given all the facts if the doctor does not feel that they will be able to fully understand their condition. There is a general acceptance among both the medical profession and the laity that it is doctors who know best in such circumstances and that the women concerned either do not need to know the full rationale behind the decision, or that they will not be able to fully understand the medical necessity for such a decision. A final factor in telling women that their labour is taking too long may be that, after a prolonged and exhausting labour, women are more likely to agree to the operation, as they can more immediately relate to what is being said, than if the doctor was to go into a long and detailed explanation about their condition.

A second explanation for the discrepancy between what women are being told and the reasons that consultants say they perform caesareans is that consultants may be reluctant to give the full information to researchers, particularly if they feel that the research may depict them in a bad light. For example, consultants may be reluctant to admit that caesareans are performed because of factors such as length of time in labour as they may then leave themselves open to criticism and accusations of performing operations to suit their own convenience and/or the use of hospital resources rather than medical necessity.

3. Fetal distress (19.8 per cent in 1996, 20.7 per cent in 1991/2)
Almost one in five women having caesarean sections were told that their babies were distressed. Fetal distress as an explanation for caesarean birth often accompanies other reasons such as labour taking too long and/or cephalopelvic disproportion. Yet interpretations of the term 'fetal distress' may differ because of the vagueness of definition. It is also clear that fetal distress is not an absolute indication for caesarean section (see Chapter 10 for discussion of indications).

4. Cephalopelvic disproportion (19.5 per cent in 1996, 28.7 per cent in 1991/2)
Almost one in five women were told that their babies were too big for their pelves in the 1996 survey. This represents a thirty per cent drop in this indication since 1991/2.

A caesarean rate of almost 20 per cent for cephalopelvic disproportion is surprising, given a caesarean rate nationally of just over 15 per cent. This means that almost three per cent of the childbearing population have babies which are considered to be too big for their pelves. It was not within the remit of this research to investigate the size of women's pelvic openings in comparison to the size of their babies, so the extent to which this is actually the case is left to speculation. However, it does appear to be unlikely that three per cent of women of childbearing age have babies that are too large for their pelves. What this may indicate therefore, is that women are being given this explanation for alternative reasons. It may be the case, for example, that rather than attempt a labour which may be problematic, the consultant decides that an elective caesarean is preferable. Similarly it could be that time can be saved if the consultant opts for an elective caesarean rather than allowing the woman a full trial of labour which may possibly end with an emergency caesarean in any case.

However, assessments of women's pelvic size are problematic. Evidence suggests that attempts to assess whether or not the baby can pass through the pelvis are unreliable predictors since some women whose pelves have been shown to be 'radiologiclly inadequate' have succeeded in giving birth vaginally. Further, women whose pelves have been assessed as 'radiologically adequate' have required emergency caesareans (Krishnamurthy et al., 1991).

5. Breech presentation (17.2 per cent in 1996, 19.0 per cent in 1991/2)
One in six caesareans were performed because of breech presentation in the 1996 survey. The 1991/2 figure represented a substantial rise in the use of caesarean section for infants presenting in breech. It appears that numbers of caesareans for this indication have remained relatively stable over the period of study.

A survey of consultants' attitudes revealed that only one in seven (14.5 per cent) had a policy of caesarean for breech presentation. Almost a third (30.8 per cent) said that it would depend on the circumstances of individual cases (Francome et al., 1993). In a smaller scale study of obstetric health care professionals' opinions on the rising caesarean section rate, 30 per cent of consultant obstetricians and eight per cent of midwives cited breech presentation as a reason for increasing rates (Francome, 1994). It is clear from the results of the current study that breech presentation is seen to justify the necessity for caesarean section in a substantial proportion of cases.

These results demonstrate that the main indicators for caesarean section, as reported by the recipients of care, were repeat operations, dystocia, fetal distress, cephalopelvic disproportion and breech presentation. However, further analysis reveals differences in the reasons according to whether there was an emergency or an elective caesarean.

REASONS FOR ELECTIVE CAESAREANS
The results show that three major indications account for the majority of elective caesareans. These are: previous caesareans, breech presentation and cephalopelvic disproportion. There has been a 50 per cent reduction in the number of elective caesareans performed for cephalopelvic disproportion over the five year period of study from 41.7 per cent to 18.9 per cent. In 1991/2 this was the second largest indicator, it is now third and breech presentation has moved into second place. Almost a half (46.2 per cent) of the elective operations were carried out because women have had previous caesareans. Almost two in seven women (28.0 per cent) were operated on because their babies were in breech position and almost one in five women (18.9 per cent) were told that their babies were too big for vaginal delivery. Lesser reasons for elective caesareans given by women under the 'other' option were previous problems with vaginal delivery including one woman who said that she had 'lost a baby by natural birth' and another who said that her 'previous delivery by forceps needed a repair a year later for bladder prolapse'. One respondent reported that her caesarean

had been elective because she 'had an eptopic pregnancy the previous year leaving my womb too weak for labour'. This group also included an assortment of other complications such as oblique presentation, placental deterioration, reduction in amniotic fluid (oligo hydramnios), previous surgery including vaginal reconstruction, bi-cornuate uterus, perforated uterus, toxaemia, fibroids, one woman who said that she was being sterilized, another who had suffered a brain haemorrhage at 18 and one spina bifida patient.

	1991/2		1996	
	n	%	n	%
repeat caesarean	75	56.8	66	46.2
breech presentation	38	28.8	40	28.0
cephalopelvic disproportion	55	41.7	27	18.9
baby was small for dates	4	3.0	11	7.7
diabetes	4	3.0	8	5.6
transverse lie	4	3.0	8	5.6
high blood pressure	0	0.0	8	5.6
maternal age	4	3.0	6	4.2
twins	2	1.5	4	2.8
placenta praevia	2	1.5	2	1.4
dystocia	3	2.3	4	2.8
cord prolapse	1	0.8	1	0.7
cord around baby's neck	2	1.5	1	0.7
antepartum haemorrhage	4	3.0	0	0.0
fetal distress	1	0.8	0	0.0
other reasons	17	12.9	27	18.9
Total no. reasons	216		213	
Average no. reasons per woman	1.6		1.5	
Total no. women	132		143	

Percentages total more than 100 as many women were given a number of reasons for their caesareans

Table 12.6: Reasons for elective caesareans, 1991/2 and 1996

REASONS FOR EMERGENCY CAESAREANS

Table 12.7 shows that there are a few major reasons that women were given for their emergency operations. The three major reasons that account for the majority of emergency operations, dystocia, fetal distress and cephalopelvic disproportion, have remained constant over the five year period of study. Women commenting on 'other' reasons for their operations identified failed induction, failed forceps, waters breaking early, perforated uterus and variations on unusual presentation as indicators.

	1991/2		1996	
	n	%	*n*	%
dystocia	71	42.3	63	38.2
fetal distress	61	36.3	61	37.0
cephalopelvic disproportion	31	18.5	33	20.0
breech presentation	19	11.3	13	7.9
antepartum haemorrhage	12	7.1	10	6.1
cord around baby's neck	11	6.5	9	5.5
repeat caesarean	12	7.1	8	4.8
transverse lie	5	3.0	6	3.6
high blood pressure	7	4.2	5	3.0
baby was small for dates	3	1.8	4	2.4
twins	1	0.6	3	1.8
maternal age	1	0.6	2	1.2
placenta praevia	1	0.6	2	1.2
diabetes	2	1.2	2	1.2
cord prolapse	2	1.2	1	0.6
other reasons	30	17.8	15	9.1
Total no. reasons	269		237	
Average no. reasons per woman	1.6		1.4	
Total no. women	168		165	

Percentages total more than 100 as many women were given a number of reasons for their caesareans

Table 12.7: Reasons for emergency caesareans, 1991/2 and 1996

Women requesting caesarean section

In an attempt to ascertain whether the increase in the use of caesarean section was due to doctors responding to women's requests, women were asked: 'Did you ask to have a caesarean section?'.

The results show that in the 1996 study over one in five women (21.3 per cent) asked for a caesarean. This represented a significant difference in the data since 1991/2 when only one in eight women (13.2 per cent) said that they had asked to have the operation (p= .05, x^2= 6.190, df= 1). The rise represents not only an increase of over 60 per cent in requests from women with previous caesareans but also an 160 per cent increase in requests from women with previous vaginal deliveries. This is an important issue and may be partly responsible for increases in caesarean rates overall. A survey of consultants' opinions on why the caesarean rate is rising identified women requesting the operation as one of the main reasons for the increase (Francome, 1994).

	Primigravidae		Previous caesarean section		Previous vaginal delivery		All groups	
1991/2	*n*	%	*n*	%	*n*	%	*n*	%
Requested C/S	11	8.0	21	21.9	7	11.5	39	13.2
Didn't request C/S	127	92.0	75	78.1	54	88.5	256	86.8
Total	138	100	96	100	61	100	295	100
1996	*n*	%	*n*	%	*n*	%	*n*	%
Requested C/S	13	8.8	27	36.5	24	30.4	64	21.3
Didn't request C/S	135	91.2	47	63.5	55	69.6	237	78.7
Total	148	100	74	100	79	100	301	100

Women who did not respond to this question are excluded from these tables

Table 12.8: Women requesting caesarean section (C/S), 1991/2 and 1996

Few primigravidae request a caesarean. The majority of women asking for the operation had previous deliveries. In 1996 one in three (36.5 per cent) women with previous caesarean asked for another. Interestingly a similar number of women with previous vaginal deliveries asked for a caesarean, presumably because of problems experienced with previous births.

Women who stated that they had requested a caesarean section were asked why. Many of the women for whom this was not the first caesarean said that they had requested the operation because the original reasons for previous caesarean were still valid. Others stressed their desire to pre-empt the need for an emergency caesarean, 'I didn't want to go through labour and end up having an emergency section like last time'. Others had requested caesareans because of concern for their babies, presumably based on their previous experiences saying for example: 'I didn't want to put baby in distress', and 'fear of baby in trouble again'. One women requested the operation because of her knowledge about her previous pregnancies:

> 'This is my fourth pregnancy, the first was delivered by forceps after a long labour, the third was caesarean. They were all large. I was scanned for size at 32 weeks, the baby was 6lb 6oz then!'

This respondent gave birth by caesarean to a 10lb 11oz baby at 39 weeks. Another woman elected to have a caesarean because she wanted more control over the situation compared to her previous section: 'My previous section was a general anaesthetic emergency. I didn't want to miss out on the birth this time. Unfortunately I have'.

This woman had a general anaesthetic for the operation following a failed attempt at spinal block. Her partner stayed with her until the general anaesthetic was administered, then had to leave.

Similarly those women who had previously given birth vaginally but had requested a caesarean for this birth stated reasons to do with their past experience(s), for example, 'previous difficult delivery'. One woman said that her,

> '... baby was in breech position. I decided this (the caesarean) was the safest way for him to be born. I also did not want to go through labour then have to have a section after all.'

Some women having their first child requested a caesarean. These were more often than not performed as an emergency after a trial of labour. 'I was in constant pain for hours and felt that I couldn't go on any longer'. One woman stated that she requested the operation because of her 'very painful labour'. Another said that she asked for a caesarean because 'I was told that forceps would be necessary and I would not agree to their use'. One respondent wanted 'to avoid a vaginal breech delivery'.

It appears, therefore, that an increasing proportion of women ask for the operation because of current or previous experiences. This means that it is very important for women to understand why the operations are being performed, to be given the appropriate information to understand what is happening to them, to be aware of the relative risks and benefits and to be enabled to make informed choices.

Type of anaesthesia for caesareans

Women were asked 'what type of anaesthesia were you given?'. The results were tabulated as follows:

	Elective				Emergency				All caesareans			
	1991/2		**1996**		1991/2		**1996**		1991/2		**1996**	
	n	%	**n**	**%**	*n*	%	**n**	**%**	*n*	%	**n**	**%**
Epidural	40	30.3	**7**	**4.9**	30	17.9	**41**	**24.9**	70	23.3	**48**	**15.6**
Spinal	35	26.5	**99**	**69.2**	9	5.4	**52**	**31.5**	44	14.7	**151**	**49.0**
General	55	41.7	**35**	**24.5**	119	70.8	**65**	**39.4**	174	58.0	**100**	**32.5**
More than 1 type	2	1.5	**2**	**1.4**	10	5.9	**7**	**4.2**	12	4.0	**9**	**2.9**
Total	132	100	**143**	**100**	168	100	**165**	**100**	300	100	**308**	**100**

Table 12.9: Type of anaesthesia for caesareans, 1991/2 and 1996

The 1991/2 data showed that almost three in five (58.0 per cent) women having caesarean sections were under general anaesthetic for the birth of their babies. The highest proportion of these being in the 'emergency' category where over two out of three (70.8 per cent) were given general anaesthesia. Even though over two out of five (41.7 per cent) women receiving elective caesareans were also under general anaesthetic at the time their babies were born, the difference between the two groups, in terms of whether local or general anaesthesia was used for their operations, was significant (p= .05, x^2= 37.969, df= 2). However, there has been a significant change in practice in the time between the two studies (p= .05, x^2= 82.623, df= 2). The 1996 data reveal a dramatic 43 per cent reduction in the use of general anaesthetic. Use of epidural anaesthetic has reduced slightly, the increase has been in the use of spinal block where the number is up 200 per cent (see Figure 12.5). Yet there remains a significant difference between the type of anaesthetic used for elective and emergency operations (p= .05, x^2= 46.898, df= 2).

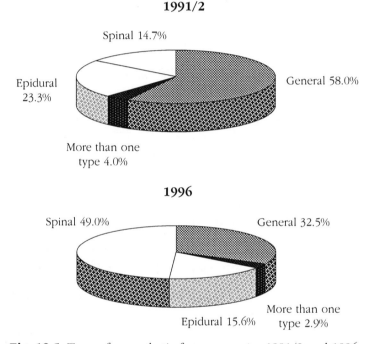

1991/2

Spinal 14.7%

Epidural 23.3%

General 58.0%

More than one type 4.0%

1996

Spinal 49.0%

General 32.5%

Epidural 15.6%

More than one type 2.9%

Fig. 12.5: Type of anaesthetic for caesareans, 1991/2 and 1996

The fact that 40 per cent of elective operations were performed with the woman under general anaesthetic in 1991/2 was a cause for concern because women were missing out on the birth of their babies and reporting negative effects postnatally. It is encouraging to see a major reduction in the use of general anaesthetic for elective caesareans as well as emergency operations. This has been matched by an increase in the use of regional anaesthetic, particularly spinal block. It is also encouraging to see that spinal block is now the most common form of anaesthetic for operations as this allows women to remain conscious and take a fuller part in the birth of their babies. This may be attributable to the increased use of spinal anaesthetic in delivery rooms generally. Therefore when the decision to perform a caesarean is made in an emergency situation, the anaesthetic is already in place.

Support during caesarean births

Women were asked 'Did you have a partner/birth companion present for the birth?'. The results were:

| | Elective | | | | Emergency | | | | All caesareans | | | |
| | 1991/2 | | 1996 | | 1991/2 | | 1996 | | 1991/2 | | 1996 | |
	n	%	*n*	%	*n*	%	*n*	%	*n*	%	*n*	%
Partner present	85	65.9	109	76.8	75	46.3	88	54.0	160	55.0	197	64.6
Partner not present	44	34.1	33	23.2	87	53.7	75	46.0	131	45.0	108	35.4
Total	129	100	142	100	162	100	163	100	291	100	305	100

Women who did not answer are excluded from this table

Table 12.10: Partners' presence during caesarean births, 1991/2 and 1996

In 1991/2 just over half (55.0 per cent) of women in the sample had their partner/birth companion present during the birth. By 1996 almost two in three (64.6 per cent) women were accompanied during their operations. This represented a significant difference in the number of women accompanied during caesareans between the 1991/2 and 1996 data (p= .05, x^2= 5.329, df= 1). The increase is evident in both the elective and emergency groups, although a significant gap remains between the two groups (1991/2: p= .05, x^2= 10.363, df= 1; 1996: p= .05, x^2= 16.226, df= 1). In 1996 three quarters (76.8 per cent) of women in the elective category had a birth companion/ partner present for their operations whereas in the emergency group just over half (54.0 per cent) were accompanied.

Many women in the emergency category commented that their partners stayed until the decision to perform the caesarean was made, or more specifically, when the general anaesthetic was administered, then partners were asked to leave. Whether or not partners are present for caesarean births is directly related to the type of anaesthesia used as Table 12.11 demonstrates.

| PARTNER PRESENT | Epidural | | | | Spinal Block | | | | General Anaesthetic | | | |
| | 1991/2 | | 1996 | | 1991/2 | | 1996 | | 1991/2 | | 1996 | |
	n	%	*n*	%	*n*	%	*n*	%	*n*	%	*n*	%
YES	56	87.5	43	93.5	45	91.8	146	96.0	59	33.7	8	7.6
NO	8	12.5	3	6.5	4	8.2	6	4.0	116	66.3	97	92.4

Women who did not answer are excluded from this table

Table 12.11: Type of anaesthesia and partners' presence at caesarean births, 1991/2 and 1996

In 1991/2 one in three (33.7 per cent) women having general anaesthetic for their caesarean sections had a partner present for the birth. This marked a change in practice and was seen as a positive trend. However, the 1996 data reveal a surprising shift whereby 92.4 per cent of women having general anaesthetic did not have a companion present for the birth. The reasons for this dramatic turnabout are not clear. The results are the same for emergency and elective caesareans and among women having general anaesthesia the proportion of elective and emergency caesareans have remained relatively static over the five year period of study. A possible explanation is that there may have been some misunderstanding about the question as some women answered 'yes' they did have a partner present but then stated 'until the general anaesthetic'. However such responses were recorded as answering 'no' as it was clear that women were not accompanied during the delivery. What is more, the question specifically asked whether women had a partner of birth companion 'present for the birth' so any misunderstanding could have only a minimal effect on the results. Further, women in both the 1991/2 and 1996 samples were asked the same question. It could therefore be expected that a similar amount of misunderstanding would occur. Such explanations clearly do not furnish the full answer for differences in the experiences of the two samples. What is clear is that whether or not women are accompanied during their caesarean deliveries is closely related to type of anaesthesia used for the operation.

Information given to women having caesareans

BEFORE THE OPERATION

Women were asked 'Before the operation were you able to find out all you wanted to know about your condition?'. The results were tabulated as follows:

	Elective				Emergency				All caesareans			
	1991/2		**1996**		1991/2		**1996**		1991/2		**1996**	
	n	%	*n*	%	*n*	%	*n*	%	*n*	%	*n*	%
YES	125	95.4	**138**	**97.2**	134	81.7	**146**	**90.1**	259	87.8	**284**	**93.4**
NO	6	4.6	**4**	**2.8**	30	18.3	**16**	**9.9**	36	12.2	**20**	**6.6**
Total	131	100	**142**	**100**	164	100	**162**	**100**	295	100	**304**	**100**

Women who answered 'don't know' to this question are excluded from the table

Table 12.12: Whether women felt that they had been adequately informed about their condition, 1991/2 and 1996

In 1991/2 a high percentage (87.8 per cent) of respondents felt that they had been kept adequately informed of their condition. However, a significant difference was found on this issue between the women who had been given emergency operations and those having elective caesareans (p= .05, x^2= 11.533, df= 1). Less than one in six (18.3 per cent) of the women receiving emergency caesareans said that they were not able to find out all they wanted to know about their condition compared with more than one in twenty (4.6 per cent) who said 'no' in the elective caesarean group. At the time I believed that this was probably due to the fact that in an emergency situation, there is not enough time to adequately inform women of all that is happening. However, in the results of the 1996 survey this discrepancy has reduced substantially showing a significant difference with the earlier data ($p= .05$, $x^2= 4.945$, $df= 1$). The number of women having emergency operations reporting that they were adequately informed about their condition has risen by ten per cent leaving a difference of only eight per cent between the two groups, a small but significant difference ($p= .05$, $x^2= 5.041$, $df= 1$). Thus it appears that even in emergency situations it is possible to inform women of what is happening. The difference in results between 1991/2 and 1996 may be due to sample differences. However, if this is not the full explanation then it may reflect a change in practice in labour wards towards ensuring women are adequately informed.

INFORMATION ABOUT TREATMENT

Women were then asked 'Were you kept informed of the treatment you were being given?'. The overwhelming response was that women felt that they had been kept informed of their treatment. In 1991/2, 95.7 per cent, and in 1996, 98.7 per cent answered 'yes' to this question. One respondent said 'every person involved in the delivery suite and operating theatre explained everything in detail, they were great'.

Some women in 1991/1 said that they had not been kept informed about their treatment. For example, one respondent would have liked to have been told 'how the pain killing treatments would have affected me'. Another simply said that she would like to have been told 'everything'. In 1996 the women who answered 'no' to this question said 'I wish I had been told that a possible side effect of spinal anaesthesia was severe throbbing headaches', 'I wanted to know why it took so long, what the problems were', 'I was unaware that the spinal was given on the actual operating table'. Another said that she had not been given enough information about treatment but that it was 'due to the drugs' rather than not being offered the information. Similarly another stated 'I was not able to understand due to my drug intake but my husband was kept informed'.

INFORMATION ABOUT THE BABY'S CONDITION

The next question was 'Do you feel that you were kept fully informed of your baby's condition?'. The overwhelming majority of women answered 'yes' to this question, in 1991/2, 91.7 per cent and 95.0 per cent in 1996. Therefore it appears that women overwhelmingly felt that they were kept fully informed of their baby's condition. Of the 17 women who answered 'no' to this question in 1991/2, the majority (12 out of 17, 70.6 per cent) were primigravidae who had emergency operations. Most of these women felt that they wanted to be better informed about their baby's condition. One woman said that she would have liked to have been told about the effects of the operation on her baby, for example, the after-effects such as shock, anaemia and jaundice. Another said that she would have liked to have been told what risk the operation would be to her baby. Other comments related to the general condition of the baby before, during, and immediately after, the operation. One woman stated that her baby's condition was never discussed. Of the 15 women who said that they were not adequately informed about their baby's condition in 1996, there were eight comments, most from primigravidae. They said that they would like to have been told 'that she (the baby) was in distress', 'if the baby was happy, heartbeat etc.', 'as much as possible', and 'everything'. One respondent complained that 'they did not keep a check on the baby', another commented that she would have liked to have been told about 'the problem with raised legs which is apparently common with breech babies, and why it occurs, how long it takes to settle etc.'. One woman appears to have had a particularly bad experience regarding information about her baby during the operation:

> 'I would have liked to have been told that the baby was okay when she was born. The doctor did not really let us know what was happening. We only knew when the baby started crying and my husband asked "is that the baby born?"'

The data show that more women answered 'no' to this question in 1991/2. It is not the case, however, that all the women who answered 'no' to this question actually wanted more information. For example, one woman said: 'I was glad not to be told the full details until the next day'. Similarly, another implied that more information would have made her feel worse, 'I was distressed and it would have upset me more if I knew baby was distressed'. Another respondent expressed feelings of wanting to know more but also accepting that such information may have had a negative effect on her, she said that she would have liked to have been told about her baby's 'position in the womb, but perhaps this would have been disheartening'.

Therefore, it appears from the results that, overall, women were increasingly satisfied with the amount of information they received from the staff in hospital.

WOMEN'S UNDERSTANDING AT THE TIME OF BIRTH

Women were asked 'At the time, did you understand why a caesarean section was needed?'. In 1991/2, 92.0 per cent of women in the sample said that they understood why their caesarean was needed. In 1996, 94.8 per cent said 'yes'. Only three per cent answered 'no' to this question in 1991/2 and 1.3 per cent in 1996. The remaining respondents said that they did not know or could not remember. This result indicates that most women felt that they understood why they had been given a caesarean. Interestingly, of the nine women in the 1996 sample who said that they could not remember if, at the time of the operation, they understood why the section was needed, eight had general anaesthetic for the surgery.

Women's post-operative experiences

DO WOMEN WHO HAVE CAESAREANS SUFFER?

Women were asked 'Do you consider that you suffered as a result of having a caesarean?'. The results were as follows:

	Elective				Emergency				All caesareans			
	1991/2		**1996**		1991/2		**1996**		1991/2		**1996**	
	n	%	*n*	%	*n*	%	*n*	%	*n*	%	*n*	%
YES	26	20.0	**22**	**15.7**	90	55.9	**31**	**19.7**	116	39.9	**53**	**17.8**
NO	104	80.0	**118**	**84.3**	71	44.1	**126**	**80.3**	175	60.1	**244**	**82.2**
Total	130	100	**140**	**100**	161	100	**157**	**100**	291	100	**297**	**100**

Women who did not answer are excluded from this table

Table 12.13: Whether women having caesareans feel that they suffer, 1991/2 and 1996

In 1991/2 three in five women (60.1 per cent) did not feel that they suffered as a result of the caesarean operation. However a significant difference existed between women giving birth by elective sections and those having emergency operations. Four in five (80.0 per cent) women who had elective caesareans did not feel that they suffered as a result of giving birth by caesarean. In contrast, almost three in five (55.9 per cent) of the women who received emergency caesareans felt that they had suffered (p= .05, x^2= 37.187, df= 1). There has been a significant change in women's perceptions of caesarean birth over the five year period of study (p= .05, x^2= 33.724, df= 1). The 1996 data show that the number of women feeling that they had suffered as a result of the operation has dropped from two in five (39.9 per cent) to almost one in six (17.8 per cent). Interestingly the gap evident in the experiences of women having elective and emergency operations in 1991/2 is not evident in the 1996 data and no significant difference was found (p= .05, x^2= 0.568, df= 1).

Comments from women about why they felt that they had suffered concentrated on: not participating in the birth of their babies; their feelings about being separated from their babies immediately after the birth; the pain of the operation; losing out on a natural birth; the lengthy recovery period; and, in particular, perceived problems with bonding. For example one woman stated, 'it is far harder than a natural birth but I had no choice'. Others mentioned that the caesarean was 'more painful' than expected and that they had suffered because of 'general discomfort and lack of mobility' (for more details on women's responses to suffering, see Chapter 13 and discussion of results).

PAIN EXPECTED BY WOMEN

It would appear that the pain women experience after the operation is perceived to be a prime source of suffering among women having caesareans. However, when asked specifically about their experience of pain (that is: 'After the caesarean section did you feel pain in the wound more or less as expected?') it does not appear that many women experienced pain more than they expected. The results were:

	Elective				Emergency				All caesareans			
	1991/2		**1996**		1991/2		**1996**		1991/2		**1996**	
	n	%	*n*	%	*n*	%	*n*	%	*n*	%	*n*	%
MORE	28	21.2	**23**	**16.2**	52	32.3	**32**	**19.7**	80	27.3	**55**	**18.1**
AS	77	58.3	**85**	**59.9**	80	49.7	**91**	**56.2**	157	53.6	**176**	**57.9**
LESS	27	20.5	**34**	**23.9**	29	18.0	**39**	**24.1**	56	19.1	**73**	**24.0**
Total	132	100	**142**	**100**	161	100	**162**	**100**	293	100	**304**	**100**

Women who did not answer are excluded from this table

Table 12.14: Women's experience of pain following caesarean birth compared to their expectations, 1991/2 and 1996

The results show that over half the women who had caesareans experienced as much pain as they had expected. The number of women experiencing more pain than expected has reduced over the five year period of study from just over one in four (27.3 per cent) to just over one in six (18.1 per cent). This reduction is evident in both elective and emergency groups. However, the number of women in the emergency category experiencing more pain than expected has reduced substantially over the five year period so that the difference between the two groups, in terms of experience of pain, has virtually disappeared.

The results were then divided into those women who had experienced previous caesareans and those who had not, to see if their expectations and experience of pain differed.

	Primigravidae				Previous caesarean(s)				Previous vaginal delivery			
	1991/2		**1996**		1991/2		**1996**		1991/2		**1996**	
	n	%	*n*	%	*n*	%	*n*	%	*n*	%	*n*	%
MORE	46	34.1	**30**	**20.6**	13	13.4	**7**	**9.4**	21	34.4	**18**	**21.4**
AS	55	40.7	**72**	**49.3**	73	75.3	**52**	**70.3**	29	47.6	**52**	**61.9**
LESS	34	25.2	**44**	**30.1**	11	11.3	**15**	**20.3**	11	18.0	**14**	**16.7**
Total	135	100	**146**	**100**	97	100	**74**	**100**	61	100	**84**	**100**

Women who did not answer are excluded from this table

Table 12.15: Previous birth experiences and expectations of pain, 1991/2 and 1996

The results show that for both 1991/2 and 1996 it is women without experience of previous caesarean deliveries that encounter more pain than expected. Not surprisingly the results show that in 1996 only one in ten (9.4 per cent) women with previous caesareans had more pain than expected, compared to one in five primigravidae and those with previous vaginal deliveries (20.6 per cent and 21.4 per cent respectively). Of women with previous caesareans, 90.6 per cent had as much or less pain than expected, presumably because of prior experience. The fact that as many as one in four women without previous caesareans had more pain than expected may point to the fact that all women need to be fully informed about caesarean birth and prepared for the after-effects.

'OTHER' POST–OPERATIVE FEELINGS

Women were asked: 'What else did you feel after the operation? They were then given a list of options: 'happy, tired, weak, relieved, sick, well, depressed, other'.

The results were:

	Elective				Emergency				Both Groups			
	1991/2		**1996**		1991/2		**1996**		1991/2		**1996**	
	n	%	***n***	**%**	*n*	%	***n***	**%**	*n*	%	***n***	**%**
Happy	–	–	**76**	**53.1**	–	–	**53**	**32.1**	–	–	**129**	**41.9**
Relieved	–	–	**80**	**55.9**	–	–	**101**	**61.2**	–	–	**181**	**58.8**
Well	–	–	**20**	**14.0**	–	–	**22**	**13.3**	–	–	**42**	**13.6**
Tired	101	76.5	**100**	**69.9**	151	89.9	**131**	**79.4**	252	84.0	**231**	**75.0**
Weak	67	50.8	**47**	**32.9**	99	58.9	**79**	**47.9**	166	55.3	**126**	**40.9**
Sick	18	13.6	**24**	**16.8**	34	20.2	**27**	**16.4**	52	17.3	**51**	**16.6**
Depressed	12	9.1	**6**	**4.2**	33	19.6	**10**	**6.1**	45	15.0	**16**	**5.2**
Total	132		**142**		168		**165**		300		**308**	

Percentages total more than 100 as some women indicated more than one response

Table 12.16: Caesarean women's post-operative feelings, 1991/2 and 1996

The 1996 data show a reduction in the number of caesarean women reporting negative post-operative feelings compared to the 1991/2 study. This may, in part, be due to modifications in the design of the questionnaire and the addition of extra categories to map women's responses. This could have had the effect of dispersing responses among a larger number of categories thus reducing the total number in each box. However, no restriction was placed on women in terms of the number of boxes they could tick and so any difference because of design modifications is likely to be minimal. The change in perceptions is more likely to be due to better experiences in the 1996 sample in terms of being better informed about caesarean birth and the reduced use of general anaesthetic in this sample. Even so, some differences are evident in the experiences of women who had elective operations and those having emergency sections in 1996. More elective caesarean women felt happy after the operation, over half (53.1 per cent) compared to a third (32.1 per cent) of emergency caesarean women. Similarly, more emergency caesarean women reported feeling weak post-operatively, almost a half (47.9 per cent) compared to a third (32.9 per cent) of women having elective operations.

Other comments that women made regarding this question reflected mostly negative feelings such as 'sore', 'shaky', 'lightheaded', 'tearful', 'confused', 'disappointed', 'cold', 'vacant', 'dizzy', 'anxious', 'cheated' and 'hungry!!!'. One woman said that she was 'in shock and resentful towards the baby for the first day'. Some women mentioned headaches or migraine and two reported 'buzzing' or 'fuzzy sensation' in the ears. One said that she felt 'fear because of the pain, worried about the baby who was taken to the SCBU and guilt because I felt no rush of love for the baby'. Others reported more positive feelings. One said that she felt 'absolutely delighted', another expressed gratitude saying that she felt 'extremely thankful that the staff were so competent and considerate in difficult circumstances'.

The mother-child relationship

SPECIAL CARE BABY UNITS (SCBU)

Women were asked: 'Was your baby taken to intensive care/Special Care Baby Unit?'. The results were:

| | Elective | | | | Emergency | | | | All caesareans | | | |
| | 1991/2 | | 1996 | | 1991/2 | | 1996 | | 1991/2 | | 1996 | |
	n	%	*n*	%	*n*	%	*n*	%	*n*	%	*n*	%
Baby went to SCBU	14	11.2	**22**	**15.5**	34	21.4	**42**	**25.6**	48	16.9	**64**	**20.9**
Baby didn't go to SBCU	111	88.8	**120**	**84.5**	125	78.6	**122**	**74.4**	236	83.1	**242**	**79.1**
Total	125	100	**142**	**100**	159	100	**164**	**100**	284	100	**306**	**100**

Women who answered 'don't know' are excluded from this table

Table 12.17: Caesarean babies taken into SCBU, 1991/2 and 1996

The results have remained constant over the five year period of study as no significant difference was found between the 1991/2 and 1996 data. They show that the majority of babies born by caesarean section were not taken into the SCBU. However a higher proportion of babies born by emergency section went into intensive care compared to those born by elective operations and the difference was found to be significant (1991/2: $p= .05$, $x^2= 4.468$, $df= 1$; 1996: $p= .05$, $x^2= 4.117$, $df= 1$). Two in three caesarean babies who went into intensive care were born by emergency operations. Furthermore, over half the caesarean babies taken into intensive care were from primigravidae (50.0 per cent in 1991/2 and 56.2 per cent in 1996), the largest proportion of these (over 80 per cent) being from emergency sections.

INCUBATORS
Women were asked 'Did your baby need to be in an incubator?'.

	Elective				Emergency				All caesareans			
	1991/2		**1996**		1991/2		**1996**		1991/2		**1996**	
	n	%	*n*	%	*n*	%	*n*	%	*n*	%	*n*	%
Needed incubation	17	13.6	**23**	**16.4**	37	24.0	**40**	**24.4**	54	19.4	**63**	**20.7**
Didn't need incubation	108	86.4	**117**	**83.6**	117	76.0	**124**	**75.6**	225	80.6	**241**	**79.3**
Total	125	100	**140**	**100**	154	100	**164**	**100**	279	100	**304**	**100**

Women who answered 'don't know' are excluded from this table

Table 12.18: Caesarean babies placed in incubators, 1991/2 and 1996

The results from both studies demonstrate that, overall, babies born by caesarean section did not need to be placed in incubators with only around one in five needing incubation. Slightly more emergency caesarean babies were placed in incubators after birth than babies from elective caesareans, one in four compared to one in six. Of the babies who went into incubators the majority (63.5 per cent) were from emergency operations.

Women who said that their babies were placed in an incubator were then asked how long their babies were in an incubator for. The mode answer to this question demonstrated that most babies were kept in incubators for up to and including one day.

HOW SOON AFTER BIRTH THE CAESAREAN MOTHERS SAW THEIR BABIES
Women were asked 'Did you see your baby as soon as she or he was born?'. The results were as follows:

	Elective				Emergency				All caesareans			
	1991/2		**1996**		1991/2		**1996**		1991/2		**1996**	
	n	%	*n*	%	*n*	%	*n*	%	*n*	%	*n*	%
Saw baby	86	66.2	**107**	**74.8**	66	39.8	**84**	**50.9**	152	51.4	**191**	**62.0**
Didn't see baby	39	30.0	**32**	**22.4**	78	47.0	**73**	**44.2**	117	39.5	**105**	**34.1**
Couldn't remember	5	3.8	**4**	**2.8**	22	13.2	**8**	**4.9**	27	9.1	**12**	**3.9**
Total	130	100	**143**	**100**	166	100	**165**	**100**	296	100	**308**	**100**

Women who did not answer this question are excluded from the table

Table 12.19: Whether caesarean mothers saw their babies immediately after the birth, 1991/2 and 1996

In 1991/2 just over half (51.4 per cent) the women in the sample saw their babies as soon as they were born. By 1996 this proportion had risen to three in five (62.0 per cent), although the difference was not found to be significant (p= .05, x^2= 3,473, df= 1). In 1991/2 only two in five (39.8 per cent) women who had emergency caesareans saw their babies immediately compared to two in three (66.2 per cent) of the elective group who did. The 1996 data reveal that the number of emergency caesarean women seeing their babies immediately after the birth rose to 50.9 per cent. However, a corresponding increase in the number of women in the elective category reporting that they saw their babies immediately after delivery means that the significant difference between the two groups highlighted by the 1991/2 data remains (1991/2: p= .05, x^2= 13.442, df=1; 1996: p= .05; x^2= 16.739, df= 1).

In 1991/2 a higher proportion of the emergency caesarean women could not remember whether or not they saw their baby as soon as it was born, 13.2 per cent compared to only 3.8 per cent of elective births who answered 'can't remember' to this question. One explanation for this was that women having emergency operations were more likely to have been given general anaesthesia and were therefore more likely to be drowsy and disorientated following the birth. This difference is not evident in the 1996 data, presumably because of the reduced use of general anaesthetic for caesarean sections.

Women who answered 'No/Can't remember' were further asked: 'How long did you have to wait?', 'Why did you have to wait?' and 'How did you feel about this?'.

Of the women who specified a time that they had to wait to see their babies for the first time in the 1996 sample, 29 women had to wait less than an hour, some for only a few minutes. Thirty one had to wait an hour or more. Ten women had to wait a day or longer. The numbers of women responding to this question were too small to demonstrate any significant differences between women having elective and those who had emergency caesareans.

The overwhelming majority of women responding to the question 'Why did you have to wait to see your baby?' said that it was because they were waiting for the effects of the general anaesthetic to wear off. The next popular answer was that the baby had difficulties or had been taken to the SCBU and, thirdly, that the mother had problems or was too ill to see the baby.

Answers to the question 'How do you feel about this?' were divided into positive, negative and neutral responses. Positive responses included feeling 'fine', 'okay' and 'pleased'. Negative responses were feeling 'confused', 'too ill', 'nothing', 'disappointed', 'sad/upset' and 'worried' or 'anxious'. Responses classified as 'neutral' included women who said that they felt 'resigned', those who did not care because they were asleep and those who said that they could not remember. The results were as follows:

	Elective				Emergency				All caesareans			
	1991/2		**1996**		1991/2		**1996**		1991/2		**1996**	
	n	%	***n***	**%**	*n*	%	***n***	**%**	*n*	%	***n***	**%**
Positive	22	75.9	**15**	**60.0**	20	42.5	**9**	**20.9**	42	55.3	**24**	**35.3**
Negative	6	20.7	**6**	**24.0**	21	44.7	**18**	**41.9**	27	35.5	**24**	**35.3**
Neutral	1	3.4	**4**	**16.0**	6	12.8	**16**	**37.2**	7	9.2	**20**	**29.4**
Total	29	100	**25**	**100**	47	100	**43**	**100**	76	100	**68**	**100**

Table 12.20: Women's feeling at not seeing their babies immediately after birth, 1991/2 and 1996

The results show that of the women who responded to this question in 1991/2 just over half (55.3 per cent) reported positive feelings about not seeing their babies as soon as they were born. By 1996 this number had dropped to one in three with only 35.3 per cent reporting positive feelings. The differences evident between the elective and emergency caesarean groups in 1991/2 are apparent in the 1996 data. Over three quarters (75.9 per cent) of women who had elective caesareans who answered this question reported positive feelings in 1991/2. By 1996 this had reduced to three in five (60.0 per cent) reporting positive feelings. However the significant difference between the elective and emergency groups has remained with more women from the emergency caesarean group reporting negative feelings towards not seeing their babies immediately after delivery in 1991/2 and 1996 (1991/2: p= .05, x^2= 8.197, df= 2; 1996: p= .05, x^2= 10.684, df= 2). This is possibly due to the fact that there was a high proportion of repeat caesarean cases in the elective category meaning that these women may be more prepared for the outcomes of operative delivery because of their previous experiences.

CAESAREAN SECTIONS AND BREASTFEEDING

Mothers were asked 'Did you want to breastfeed your baby?'. The results were as follows:

BREASTFEEDING	Elective				Emergency				All caesareans			
	1991/2		**1996**		1991/2		**1996**		1991/2		**1996**	
	n	%	***n***	**%**	*n*	%	***n***	**%**	*n*	%	***n***	**%**
Wanted to	62	48.1	**81**	**56.6**	89	54.9	**102**	**61.8**	151	51.9	**183**	**59.4**
Didn't want to	60	46.5	**53**	**37.1**	62	38.3	**55**	**33.3**	122	41.9	**108**	**35.1**
Unsure	7	5.4	**9**	**6.3**	11	6.8	**8**	**4.9**	18	6.2	**17**	**5.5**
Total	129	100	**143**	**100**	162	100	**165**	**100**	291	100	**308**	**100**

Women who did not answer this question are excluded from the table

Table 12.21: Whether caesarean-delivered women wanted to breastfeed, 1991/2 and 1996

The results revealed that in 1991/2 over half (51.9 per cent) the women in the sample said that they wanted to breastfeed. By 1996 this number had risen to 59.4 per cent of women. Over two in five (41.9 per cent) said that they did not want to breastfeed their baby in 1991/2, this went down to one in three (35.1 per cent) in 1996, suggesting that breastfeeding was more popular overall among caesarean delivered women in the 1996 sample than it was is 1991/2. The difference, however, was not found to be significant (p= .05, x^2= 3.041, df= 1).

Women who said that they did not want to breastfeed were then asked why this was. In 1991/2 the majority (73.0 per cent) said that their decision not to breastfeed stemmed from their being 'not too keen on breastfeeding'. By 1996 only half (50.0 per cent) gave this explanation. Instead, women cited wanting to share the feeding and preferring bottle feeding as reasons for not breastfeeding their babies in 1996. Eleven per cent said that they had 'changed their mind' about breastfeeding in 1991/2, 9.3 per cent said this in 1996. In 1991/2, 13.1 per cent said that they did not want to breastfeed because they 'felt too ill', 8.3 per cent cited this reason in 1996.

No significant differences emerged between the elective and emergency caesarean groups in terms of wanting to breastfeed (1991/2: p= .05, x^2= 1.487, df=1; 1996: p= .05, x^2= 0.454, df= 1). Further, similar reasons were given by women in each group for not breastfeeding, apart from women who said that they preferred bottle feeding or had experienced previous failure in breastfeeding whereby many more were in the elective caesarean category. This is to be expected due to the higher number of women with previous deliveries in this group.

Further reasons given by women for not wanting to breastfeed in 1996 were that they had 'inverted nipples', because they felt that breastfeeding was inconvenient, or they suffered with breast abscesses. Two women from the elective caesarean group said that they did not want to breastfeed because of older children at home and their desire to share their time. One said that she could not breastfeed because of her diabetes. Three women in the sample said that they would not breastfeed because they had twins and five women were worried about the effect that drugs given to them would have on their breastmilk and therefore their babies. One respondent stated that she was 'advised not to, due to medication'.

Women's responses to the question on breastfeeding in 1991/2 raised a number of concerns over the effect that the caesarean operation had on women's ability to breastfeed. The 1996 questionnaire was therefore amended to include a question on this. Women were asked: 'Do you feel that the caesarean has had an effect on your ability to breastfeed your baby?'.

The results were as follows:

	Elective		Emergency		Total	
	n	%	*n*	%	*n*	%
YES	21	14.7	32	19.4	53	17.2
NO	114	79.7	110	66.7	224	72.7
DON'T KNOW	8	5.6	23	13.9	31	10.1
Total	143	100	165	100	308	100

Table 12.22: Whether women feel that caesarean birth has an effect on their ability to breastfeed, 1996

The data reveal that a substantial proportion of women delivering by caesarean feel that the operation affects their ability to breastfeed their babies. One in six (17.2 per cent) answered 'yes' to this question. No significant difference was found in the responses of women having elective or emergency operations (p= .05, x^2= 1.751, df= 1). In commenting on why caesareans affect breastfeeding the majority of women pointed to pain and discomfort: 'a little difficult to get into position with the wound'; 'it is more difficult and painful holding the baby whilst breastfeeding'; 'positions for breastfeeding are more difficult to find'; 'lifting and positioning of baby is very difficult. I need assistance'; 'having him on me hurts my wound'. Some women mentioned that the milk had taken longer to 'come in'. Others blamed the difficulty on the anaesthetic: 'the first feed was difficult because of the general anaesthetic'. One respondent said: 'being a major operation it takes you a long time to recover and to cope with the demands of breastfeeding'. Another stated: 'I am in more pain so less patient with the baby'. Some respondents who had wanted to breastfeed said that they were unable to because of feeling too ill post-operatively. One said that she 'did not attempt to as I felt too ill, I could not cope with another complication'. Another said 'I was too ill to keep up with the demand'. One stated that she had 'too many emotions to continue breastfeeding'. Only three women blamed failure to breastfeed on the effects of caesarean section on the condition of the baby.

CAESAREAN SECTION AND BONDING

Responses to the questionnaire in 1991/2 raised concerns due to women's perceived effect of caesarean birth on their ability to bond with their babies. The 1996 questionnaire was therefore amended to include a question which directly addressed this issue. The women were asked 'Do you feel that the caesarean has had an effect on your ability to bond with your baby?'.

	Elective		Emergency		Total	
	n	%	*n*	%	*n*	%
YES	8	5.7	27	16.5	35	11.5
NO	133	94.3	137	83.5	270	88.5
Total	141	100	164	100	305	100

Women who did not answer are excluded from this table

Table 12.23: Whether women feel that caesarean birth affects their ability to bond with their babies, 1996

Overall, one in ten women (11.5 per cent) in the sample felt that the operation had an effect on their ability to bond with their babies. Although no significant difference was found between women who had elective caesareans and those who had emergency operations (p= .05, x^2= 0.041, df= 1), more emergency caesarean women felt that bonding was affected, compared to those who had elective operations (16.5 per cent and 5.7 per cent respectively). This is likely to be due to the inclusion of repeat caesareans in the elective category and again points to the fact that women need to be fully informed and prepared for the after-effects of caesarean birth.

Women who said that they felt the caesarean had had an effect on their ability to bond with their babies were asked 'in what ways?'. The majority of responses centred around the women's pain and discomfort following the operation which reduced their mobility and ability to care for their infants or simply made them feel too ill. The women said: 'I felt too ill to want to hold my baby', and 'I have not been able to do anything for her e.g. feeding, changing or cuddling'. Also women felt that bonding was affected because of 'not being able to care for the baby due to discomfort', 'because I can not look after baby', 'can not pick up the baby properly and do everything straight away', 'not being able to hold the baby', 'I can not hold him or feed him or be next to him'. Another said 'I felt no rush of love for the baby, therefore bonding was delayed for five days'. One respondent said that she had 'missed out on the first two days because of the drip etc. It was only because the staff kept bringing him in that I began to be interested'. General anaesthetic also seems to have an effect. One respondent stated that bonding was affected because of 'not being awake to see her born'. One simply said 'I felt helpless'.

These results are a cause for concern, almost one in six emergency caesarean women and one in 20 women having elective sections felt that the operation had an effect on their ability to bond with their babies. Considering the evidence available on possible long term effects of caesarean birth on the mother-child relationship in general and child development in particular (see Chapter 11), it is clear that more research is required in this area.

Conclusion

The results of this research spanning five years of study demonstrate that certain aspects of maternity services are changing with regards to caesarean birth. The ratio of emergency to elective operations have remained constant. The vast differences in the experiences of women in these two groups identified in the 1991/2 study have diminished in many cases, with less emergency caesarean women reporting negative sequelae following the operation. It appears, therefore, that much has been done in the time between the studies to improve women's experiences of caesarean birth and ensure a better outcome for the women concerned.

The greater use of general anaesthetic for caesarean sections evident in the results of the 1991/2 study was seen to be instrumental in women's negative experiences. The reduction in the use of general anaesthetic for caesarean sections evident in the 1996 data appears to have contributed significantly to women's better experiences of the operation. However, differences are still apparent in the experiences and post-operative attitudes of women having emergency caesareans and those who have elective operations. In addition, the 1996 study has highlighted a number of issues of major concern. First, more women are requesting the operation. Secondly, partners are being excluded from delivery by the continued use of general anaesthesia. Thirdly, caesarean section affects women's decisions about breastfeeding and fourthly, one in ten caesarean women feel that the operation has an effect on their ability to bond with their infants.

Clearly, hospital services have moved on since the 1991/2 study was undertaken. It is also clear that there is still much that can be achieved to ensure the best possible outcome for women who need to deliver by caesarean section.

CHAPTER THIRTEEN

Women's Experience Of Caesarean Birth

Part II: Discussion

Hypothesis One stated that caesarean birth denies women the opportunity to have a satisfying experience of childbirth and increases their suffering.

The research question was, therefore, do women suffer as a result of caesarean section?

Do women having caesareans suffer?

There is a wealth of evidence to suggest that women who have caesareans suffer negative effects both physiologically, in terms of increased rates of morbidity, and psychologically with emotions such as depression, anxiety, disappointment, guilt, lower self-esteem, inadequacy and sense of failure. What is more, caesarean delivered women have been found to report less satisfaction with the birth experience than those who deliver vaginally (see Chapter 11).

Yet the current research found that the majority of women in the samples did not feel that they had suffered as a result of the operation. This suggests that the first hypothesis has not been proved. However, there may be a number of factors at work here. First, the women in the studies were completing their questionnaires whilst in hospital at the request of the medical staff. In this position they may not have felt that they could express dissatisfaction with their treatment or care, as this could be construed as a complaint against those caring for them. As the women were still reliant on the help of others, they may have believed that it was not in their interest to suggest that they had suffered as a result of their treatment. Whilst the covering letter issued with the questionnaires stressed that the research was independent of the hospital, some women may not have acknowledged this distinction. One woman actually wrote a 'thank you' note to staff on the reverse side of the covering letter indicating that the relationship between the hospital and the research may not have been clear in the minds of some respondents.

Secondly, the power relationship between women and their doctors is such that women may not have felt dissatisfaction, believing that their caesareans were necessary, life-saving operations, and that they had only arrived at a successful outcome (the birth of their babies) with the help, knowledge and expertise of the doctors. As such, they would not feel that they had suffered as a result of having caesarean sections.

Thirdly, women may be reluctant to say that they have suffered in childbirth, which, after all, is a natural event during which most women experience some suffering. It may be perceived as a sign of weakness to admit that you have suffered and may cast doubt on your ability to fulfill your expectations of motherhood and society's expectations of you as a woman. As such, women may not acknowledge the pain, discomfort and psychological sequelae of childbirth as 'suffering'.

Despite the fact that women say they do not suffer, the comments made by women about giving birth by caesarean make it clear that many do actually suffer because of the operation, even when they may not subjectively perceive this to be the case.

Pain

The overwhelming majority of comments on a particular issue made by women who had caesareans related to the pain of the operation.

> 'I would much prefer a normal birth as the pain you have is over. But with caesarean you seem to have quite a bit of pain and discomfort for quite a while after. Also it takes you a lot longer to get back to normal which I shall find very hard.'

> 'I had a 14 hour labour and have at this stage endured a further week of pain and discomfort. I cannot sit down or stand with the baby in my arms, I have to have him reached to me and it's very frustrating.'

Women who had experienced previous vaginal deliveries felt that the pain of caesarean section was particularly worthy of comment, 'Much less enjoyable and more painful than a natural birth' and 'my natural labour was less painful'.

Many women felt that the post-operative pain adversely affected their ability to cope with their newborn babies. One woman said that she had suffered 'because of not being able to see my baby properly as I was very sore and couldn't manoeuvre the same'. Another commented that her suffering had been caused by 'the pain after and inability to move and deal with my baby straight away'.

It is astonishing that women are so surprised by the pain of a caesarean section which, after all, is a major abdominal surgical operation. But not so surprising when considering the prevailing idea that the caesarean is a painless way to give birth, that women who have caesareans have somehow taken the 'soft' option and not had to suffer the intensity of the pain of labour. One woman said:

'It is annoying that other Mums think you've had an easy time without the labour etc., but it is really hard getting yourself pulled together afterwards.'

It appears that there is a general lack of understanding among women about exactly what caesarean birth entails and the length of time that it can take to recover. Many women who have caesareans feel angry about this lack of information and the response that they get from other women.

'Myself and other women who have had babies by caesareans feel very annoyed when people who had normal deliveries think we were lucky and had an 'easy way out' as recovery is very long and painful. It is many months before you feel well again.'

The results of the current study demonstrate that women who have second or third caesareans are more prepared for abdominal delivery and therefore do not experience such severe after-effects. For example, they do not experience as much pain. One woman who had experienced a previous caesarean found that the second operation was not as painful as the first:

'The first section was very painful and I was shocked at the severity of it. With the second one I was a bit wary because I knew of the pain I was in with the first. But it was nowhere near as bad.'

Others find that a second or third caesarean is less traumatic:

'With the first caesarean there was great disappointment and feeling that I had suffered a labour for nothing. This time I was fairly optimistic about delivering normally but knew there was the possibility of a second caesarean. Therefore I don't feel so let down this time.'

This may indicate that a degree of preparation and knowing what to expect decreases negative physiological sequelae. While women perceive that they have been adequately informed it is clear that many are inadequately prepared. Many are shocked or surprised at the intensity of the pain experienced which could indicate a lack of information and therefore preparation amongst women having caesareans. One in six women in the 1996 sample felt more pain than they expected. This represents a drop from one in four of the 1991/2 sample and may therefore suggest that hospital staff are preparing women for the after-effects or that there is more information on caesarean birth available generally. But there is still some way to go. The fact that so many women felt that their experience of pain was worthy of note and comment indicates a level of suffering among caesarean patients.

Not being able to give birth naturally

There is evidence to suggest that caesarean mothers feel disappointment or anger at not being able to give birth naturally or being 'cheated' of a vaginal delivery. Women may not construe disappointment and sense of failure as indications of suffering but it is clear from the results of the current study that many women do suffer these emotions.

Many caesarean women feel a severe sense of loss at not being able to give birth naturally. One woman who had an elective caesarean said that she felt that she had suffered 'because of a mixture of short notice and hopes of natural childbirth that made it a traumatic experience'. Another felt 'cheated out of being able to have a normal birth'. Similarly one respondent said that she felt 'cheated because of having gone in expecting a normal delivery'.

Comments from women who had emergency caesareans include a respondent who felt that she had 'lost out on being able to deliver normally'. Even when understanding the necessity of the operation in their own case, some women still felt a severe sense of loss.

> 'It felt safer for me and baby at the time, although I am still upset that I was not able to see natural birth through.'

From these comments it is clear that women do suffer a sense of loss at not being able (or allowed) to give birth naturally and that many are angry and disappointed that they have not delivered vaginally, to the extent that they do not feel that they have given birth.

Lengthy recovery period

It appears that an important side-effect of caesarean birth that can be overlooked by the medical professions and women having babies is the lengthy recovery period associated with abdominal delivery. This may be due to a failure to perceive caesarean section as major surgery instead of simply an alternative form of childbirth. The use of language is crucial here. The fact that the procedure is called the 'caesarean section' rather than the 'caesarean operation' or 'caesarean surgery' suggests that the operation is conceptualized in a different way to other forms of surgery and this may have an effect on the way that caesarean sections are seen to affect patients compared to other forms of surgery (Oakley and Richards, 1990). Evidence from the current study supports this:

> 'Caesareans should be termed as normal operations... All along I thought a caesarean wasn't a big deal. I was told how it is done but not how you feel afterwards.'

What this means is that the expectation of a caesarean patient, from both the health care professionals and the women themselves, may be akin to the expectations of women giving birth vaginally, rather than the expectations of patients undergoing major abdominal surgery. Women may therefore expect to be able to cope with the care of their newborn infant and are treated as though they ought to be able to take the main responsibility for care. This leads to feelings of disappointment and frustration when women are not able to fulfill their expectations due to the debilitating effects of major surgery. This observation is supported by the comments from women in the current study where many felt that the lengthy recovery period following a caesarean worthy of note:

> 'I can remember sitting crying because I could not do much for him. I was stuck in bed with a drip and catheter and he was crying. It was so frustrating.'

Others said:

> 'By the second day I was up, and doing nearly everything by the third day, which caused me stress because I couldn't quite manage because of the pain I was in. It left me feeling inadequate as a mother, and I wanted to do more.'

> 'Having given birth normally the first time, this section was certainly different and I would rather have a normal birth because you can move around a lot more soon after, where with a section moving is difficult at first.'

The fact that women do not expect to be immobilized by major surgery confirms that caesarean section is conceptualized differently from other forms of surgery. This increases women's anxiety and sense of frustration. One woman said: 'After a trouble free pregnancy it is difficult to accept being "invalid" and dependent on others'. Similarly it is clear that the long recovery period following the caesarean has an adverse effect on women, especially when they have other children to think about.

> 'I had hoped to recover from this birth much more quickly than last time, whereas now presumably it will be as before, but harder, thanks to a two-year old!'

The misconception over caesarean birth points to two issues. First that women, on the whole, are unprepared for abdominal delivery and do not know what to expect, and secondly, this lack of knowledge and preparedness leads to increased suffering among caesarean patients.

Evidence from this study demonstrates therefore that women do suffer as a result of caesarean sections. Women may not perceive their bad experiences to have a lasting effect. One respondent stated:

> 'Although I found the experience of caesarean section to be traumatic because I had a short time to prepare mentally, the pain I felt afterwards, particularly on the first night, the slower recovery time, delay in bonding and the inconvenience of being unable to drive for six weeks, I feel it is a mistake to be fixated on the birth. The most important thing to me was, and always will be, a healthy baby. For me, a natural childbirth would have been an added bonus but no more than that.'

However, there is no reason to expect that negative feelings about the birth will be short-lived as the results of other studies highlight the fact that women's feelings about their childbirth experiences may have an impact on their perceived maternal roles and ultimately, their relationships with their children (Affonso and Stichler, 1978; Marut and Mercer, 1979; Trowell, 1986; Tulman, 1986; Hillan, 1992).

Emergency operations and general anaesthesia

The present study found that over half the caesareans in the sample were emergency operations. The 1991/2 study demonstrated that over 60 per cent of caesareans were performed with the patient under general anaesthesia. This raised a number of concerns because much of the negative sequelae experienced by caesarean-delivered women could be attributed to the use of general anaesthetic. However, the 1996 data reveal that the use of general anaesthetic for caesarean section reduced substantially to one in three. The majority of women receiving general anaesthesia were in the 'emergency' category in 1991/2 and this ratio remained constant over the five year period of study. That is, of women having general anaesthetic for caesarean birth, two in three were emergency cases.

The evidence available on the after-effects of caesarean birth demonstrate that the two factors associated with increased suffering among women are emergency rather than elective operations and the use of general anaesthesia (see Chapter 11).

The results of the 1991/2 study certainly supported this view with women who had general anaesthesia and emergency operations consistently reporting much higher rates of dissatisfaction and suffering postnatally. The 1996 data demonstrates improvements in women's experiences of caesarean birth across the board. Differences between women having emergency and those who have elective operations have diminished and in some cases disappeared. For example, when asked whether they felt that they had been adequately informed about their condition, 93 per cent of caesarean-delivered women said 'yes' in the 1996 study, an improvement on 88 per cent who said 'yes' in the earlier study. The largest improvement, however, was in perceptions of women in the emergency caesarean category, to the extent that there was less of a discrepancy between the experiences of women in the emergency and elective caesarean groups than identified in the 1991/2 data, in terms of whether women felt that they had been adequately informed.

Similarly, when women were asked specifically whether they felt that they had suffered as a result of having a caesarean, the overwhelming majority of women said 'no'. However, the 1991/2 data highlighted a difference of 35.9 per cent between the experiences of women having emergency caesarean and those who had elective operations, with the emergency caesarean women reporting higher levels of perceived suffering. In 1996, overall levels of reported suffering were down to 17.8 per cent from 39.9 per cent in 1991/2. The greatest improvement was in the perceptions of women in the emergency category so that differences between women in the two groups were not visible in the 1996 data.

Further, there was an overall reduction in women reporting more pain than expected after the operation. The reduction was greatest among women having emergency operations, therefore differences between emergency caesarean women and those who had elective sections identified in the 1991/2 data had virtually disappeared by 1996.

There is evidence to suggest that the experiences of women having emergency operations are improving and that the gap in experience between emergency caesarean women and those who have elective operations may be closing. Unfortunately, however, there are aspects of emergency caesarean birth that are still preventing the best possible outcome in terms of women's experience of caesarean birth.

The results of the current study show that women who have emergency operations reported negative feelings such as tiredness and weakness post-operatively more than women who had elective caesareans. Women who had elective sections reported post-operative feelings of happiness more than women who had emergency caesareans. There are a number of possible explanations for these findings.

The unexpected caesarean birth

The results of the current study are consistent with a wealth of evidence demonstrating that women who have emergency caesareans have less positive perceptions of the delivery than those who have elective operations (Cranley et al., 1983; Fawcett et al., 1992). This evidence suggests that the unexpected nature of the unplanned caesarean delivery influences women's feelings about the birth and may lead to increased suffering. This is probably because the emergency caesarean patient will usually have expected a normal delivery.

In the results of the 1991/2 study, nearly four times as many women having emergency caesareans felt that they were not kept fully informed of their condition and that of their about-to-be born baby compared to women having elective operations. At that time indications pointed to women not being adequately informed, possibly due to lack of time in the emergency situation. This was certainly the feeling amongst women having emergency operations in the sample.

> 'Obviously because I had an emergency caesarean, the after-effects were not known. Presumably these are fully discussed with a planned caesarean. I felt unable to move or cuddle baby, because I was weak, tired and upset. I felt quite ill and in pain.'

> 'I knew nothing about a caesarean birth and there wasn't enough time to explain the procedure.'

Others suggested that women need to be better prepared for the possibility of caesarean birth:

> 'I think that much more should be taught about caesareans at antenatal classes to prepare women for the after-effects of a caesarean as it seems commonplace nowadays.'

> 'I think all the information and advice you can be given by staff, doctors etc. helps immensely with both the operation and what the after-effects will be. This being so, there would be no great shocks.'

> 'It would have been better if I was more prepared for it.'

Women who had elective caesareans did not report such negative feelings:

> 'Being an elective section, I found I was much better prepared physically and mentally than my first section. Recovery from an elective section was speedier and not as traumatic to both myself and baby.'

It is therefore feasible to suggest that the unplanned and unexpected nature of emergency caesarean sections lead to increased suffering amongst women.

Results from the 1996 survey suggest however that there may be time, even in an emergency situation, for women to be fully informed. The overwhelming majority of women from both elective and emergency caesarean categories said that they had been adequately informed about their condition. One emergency caesarean respondent added 'The decision to do the caesarean section took one and a half hours only. Everything was explained'.

However, some women require more information and are unhappy that they did not receive the details that they required from hospital staff before the delivery. One respondent who had an emergency caesarean reported a traumatic experience that could have been averted by information prenatally.

> 'When they were finishing stitching, I started to be sick and then felt like I could not get any air into my lungs, as though someone was sitting on my chest. This lasted for three hours. When talking to the doctor a couple of days later she assured me that this was entirely clinical, to do with my blood pressure and temperature, and that this was quite common. Talking to other caesarean women on the wards later, we had all experienced this to some degree and felt that if we had been told this may happen beforehand then we would not have panicked as much at the time.'

Some women from the elective caesarean group were equally dissatisfied. One said:

> 'I did not anticipate so much tugging and pulling. I did not know how I would be stitched up or stapled. The number of people around me was disquieting.'

It therefore appears that although the majority of women in the studies were happy with the amount of information that they received from hospital staff, there are deficiencies in some areas with regards to informing women about procedures for caesarean birth and preparing them for the after-effects. Whether it is lack of time that prevents the appropriate information being imparted to women, or personnel or procedural restrictions within the hospital setting, is open to debate. It is unlikely, though, that even in an emergency situation, there would not be time to inform women about the operation. Lack of time, however, does appear to have an effect on women's ability to adjust mentally and prepare for caesarean birth.

More emergency caesarean women reported feelings of 'shock' as a cause of suffering following caesarean section. In explaining why they felt they had suffered as a result of the operation many emergency caesarean women stated for example, 'short notice made it a traumatic experience' and 'it was a shock'. Others said 'I found the experience of caesarean section to be traumatic because I had a short time to prepare mentally' and 'I had such short notice because of the emergency section so it never really sunk in what was happening'. It may therefore be that lack of time is a problem in relation to women coming to terms with what is happening in the emergency situation rather than staff not having time to keep women fully informed.

Participation in the birth

It appears that being awake for a caesarean operation is analogous to participating in delivery for many women. Thus women who have elective operations using regional anaesthesia do not suffer as much as those having emergency sections under general anaesthetic.

> 'My first section was done under a general anaesthetic and the second under spinal. I felt so much better and brighter in myself after the spinal. I could still feel involved in the birth, have my partner present and see my baby as soon as she was born.'

> 'I am pleased that I was able to have this operation under epidural rather than a general anaesthetic. Thus allowing me to see the baby earlier and be part of the birth process.'

If, as the evidence suggests, participation in the delivery of the baby is a critical element in perceptions of childbirth, this means that the continued over-use of general anaesthesia for caesarean section is actively denying women the ability to feel as though they have participated in the birth of their infants and may therefore lead to feelings of disappointment. The findings of the current study are consistent with this view. One respondent said: 'I felt like a failure. I was very disappointed at not being awake for the delivery'. Another commented that she had suffered 'mentally because I wanted to witness the birth'.

Hospital practice regarding the use of general anaesthetic for caesarean section is clearly changing. A reduction in its use from 58 per cent of the sample in 1991/2 to 32.5 per cent of sections performed with the woman under general anaesthetic in the 1996 study. It is also clear that health professionals are actively encouraging women to have caesareans under regional anaesthetic. For example, one respondent in the 1996 sample reported that:

> 'With chronic back stiffness I have been frightened for years of the idea of an epidural or spinal. I initially wanted a general anaesthetic. The anaesthetist persuaded me spinal was better for the baby. I was very pleased with the result – it worked very well.'

The value of regional anaesthesia for caesarean birth is well established, not just for the baby as in the example given above, but also for the woman's overall experience of the delivery. However, one in three caesareans in the current study were performed with the woman asleep under general anaesthetic, 65 per cent of these operations were emergency sections. The value of general anaesthetic in such cases is not always apparent. It is possible that in many cases where the caesarean follows a trial of labour a form of regional anaesthetic may already be in place.

It appears therefore that the needs of women may not be taken into account when decisions are made about anaesthesia for caesarean operations. Rather, decisions are based on consultant preference and/or policy, use of available resources and out-dated practices which are denying women a fulfilling start to motherhood and may have long-term detrimental effects on their relationships with their children.

Missing out on the first moments after the birth

Women who have general anaesthesia for their caesareans miss out on the first minutes, and occasionally hours, after the birth of their babies. This is a problem because not only does it affect the women's psychological state, but may have a detrimental effect on important aspects of mother/child interaction, such as bonding and breastfeeding. Women who have spinal or epidural anaesthesia do not suffer in this way.

> 'It's much better if you stay awake, there's no more pain and you get to see your baby straight away.'

However, women who are asleep when their babies are delivered miss out on those first few minutes. This may not be very important to hospital staff in terms of the daily management of business but is very important to the women concerned.

> 'This is the second time by caesarean. The first was by general anaesthetic. Last time I felt cheated that I missed so much and did not see my baby properly until the next day. This time by spinal block was wonderful, we both saw him straight away and did not miss anything.'

> 'I found the epidural better as you can see baby straight away. The first time (under general anaesthetic) I lost that bond with the baby, I didn't feel he was mine.'

> 'With having a general, I feel I missed out on the first moments.'

One woman summed up her feelings very succinctly, 'One hour recovering from anaesthetic, precious moments lost forever'.

What this points to is the differing perceptions of what the experience of childbirth should be. In Chapter 8, I suggested that there is a conflict between lay and professional views on childbirth. The results of this study are consistent with this contention and the results of previous studies (Graham and Oakley, 1981; Sargent and Stark, 1987). A successful outcome for the professionals may mean the birth of a healthy baby. Clearly this is also important for women, as some respondents demonstrated, 'The pain and discomfort seem a small price to pay for a healthy baby'. But success in childbirth may mean more in terms of a personally satisfying experience which leads to a sense of accomplishment and not to a sense of failure and loss of control.

'I felt that I was not in control of my body for the first few days. This was a lot for me to cope with.'

The use of general anaesthesia for caesarean section is denying women the ability to participate in the delivery of their children and removing them, mentally if not physically, from the experience of childbirth.

Separation of mother and baby after birth

Evidence shows that many women who deliver by caesarean are separated from their infants immediately after birth and that this early separation can have a significant impact on the subsequent relationship between mother and child (NIH, 1981; Huntingford, 1985; Hillan, 1992).

The results of the current study demonstrate that the majority of women in the sample saw their babies as soon as they were born. However an important variable affecting whether women were separated from their babies following delivery was whether or not they had emergency operations. The 1991/2 data demonstrated that more than two in three (66.2 per cent) women who had elective caesareans saw their babies immediately, whereas less than two in five (39.8 per cent) of the women who had emergency caesareans did. This gave a collective result of just over half (51.4 per cent) of the women in the sample seeing their babies as soon as they were born. This situation has improved slightly. The 1996 data revealed that 62.0 per cent of women saw their babies as soon as they were born. However, the differences identified between the elective and emergency caesarean groups in 1991/2 were evident in the 1996 results where almost three in four (74.8 per cent) women in the elective category saw their babies, but only half the women in the emergency caesarean group (50.9 per cent) experienced early postpartum contact.

Another worrying fact about emergency caesareans is the practice of routinely taking babies into intensive care units regardless of medical necessity or the condition of the child at birth. Two in three (65.6 per cent) caesarean babies who were taken to intensive care were from emergency operations. Obviously the emergency situation means that staff had cause for concern about the infant and therefore babies may need to be checked before returning to the mothers. However evidence suggests that such practices are also based on hospital routine and policy regarding emergency caesareans. This will inevitably have an effect on the mother's experience of the birth and may point to services based on routine policy rather than maternity services based on the needs of women and what is best for them and their babies.

Given the evidence demonstrating that early and continued contact between mother and child is important for the development of the relationship between the two, women who have caesareans, and in particular those who have emergency operations, together with general anaesthetic, may suffer adverse effects on their relationships with their children.

Bonding

Unequivocal evidence linking early contact between mother and child postpartum with successful bonding has been available for many years (Klaus and Kennel, 1982). The results of the current study demonstrating the frequent separation of mother and baby following emergency caesarean sections bring into question such routine practices.

What is worrying about this evidence is that the reasoning behind the immediate separation of mother and child, as well as the rationale for emergency operations and the use of general anaesthesia, is not always based on medical necessity. Therefore women's relationships with their children, and the long-term development of those children, may be put in jeopardy for such extraneous rationale as consultant preference and hospital policy, the need for services to be seen to be fully utilized, staff convenience and fear of litigation.

Results of this study show that it is the women having emergency caesareans who feel that caesarean birth has an effect on their ability to bond with their babies. However, it is not so much early separation that women point to but rather the pain and lack of mobility that women cite as affecting the bonding process.

When asked why they felt that caesareans affected their ability to bond with their babies, the respondents in this study said: 'I could not get up to her when she cried and had to rely on the midwives for help', 'I can not do much for him because of the pain', 'I felt too ill to want to hold my baby'. One respondent said that bonding was affected because of 'not being able to care for baby due to discomfort'. Another reported:

> 'When they took me back to the ward after the operation, they brought the baby in and I just said "get him out of here". I feel really guilty about my feeling towards him on that first day now, especially after seeing other women on the wards caring for their babies straight away. It was only when I realized that my baby was covered in a bad rash and needed nursing without a nappy on that I got protective towards him and then I knew I could care for him more than anyone else.'

Such comments, together with data from this study demonstrating that one in ten caesarean-delivered women feel that the operation has an effect on their ability to bond with their babies, is a cause for concern. With the current escalating caesarean section rate, a conservative estimate would conclude that 1.5 to two per cent of childbearing women may be prevented from bonding appropriately with their babies because of caesarean sections, some of which may not have been necessary. Further research into the effects of caesarean section on the mother-child relationship and long term child development is needed.

Breastfeeding

The evidence on the relationship between caesarean birth and breastfeeding is inconclusive, but some studies have shown that women who have caesareans are less likely to breastfeed than those who deliver vaginally. More specifically, it has been suggested that women who have caesareans under general anaesthesia are less likely to breastfeed than those whose operations are performed under regional anaesthetic (see Chapter 11). The results of the 1991/2 study supported this. Of the women who said that they did not want to breastfeed their babies, a higher proportion of women who had had emergency operations said that this was because they had 'changed their mind'. Obviously it could not be deduced from these data whether the women had changed their minds as a result of the operation or for some other reason. But, significantly, a further one in five (22.6 per cent) emergency caesarean women said that they did not want to breastfeed in 1991/2 because they 'felt too ill' compared to only one in thirty (3.3 per cent) of women having elective operations who gave this as a reason for not breastfeeding their babies. However, there was a much higher proportion of women who had general anaesthetic for their caesareans in the 1991/2 sample. This may account for some of the post-operative morbidity.

The 1996 data do not reveal such differences between the two groups and could therefore support findings of earlier studies which suggest that birth experiences affect breastfeeding outcomes less than pre-existing attitudes (Janke, 1988; Kearney et al., 1990). This is not to suggest that caesarean birth does not have an effect on breastfeeding outcomes, clearly it does. One in six women in the 1996 sample said that they felt this to be the case. They commented: 'I felt too ill to even try to breastfeed the baby', 'My tummy is very sore so I am unable to get into a comfortable position to breastfeed', 'I was in too much pain to sit up and feed the baby', 'I felt very sore and weak so found it hard to stay awake to feed' and 'The way I feel I just felt bottle feeding would be easiest'.

Therefore it is clear that caesarean section does have an effect on women's decisions regarding whether or not to breastfeed their babies. The recognition of the importance of breastmilk has led to the recommendation that all babies should be exclusively breastfed for the first four to six months (Royal College of Midwives, 1991). Not only because breastfeeding is best for the baby but also because it helps the uterus to return to its normal size more quickly. Yet the routine separation of mother and baby following caesareans in many cases, particularly emergency operations, coupled with the pain, discomfort, drowsiness and often feelings of sickness following general anaesthesia mean that many caesarean-delivered women are either being denied a successful start to breastfeeding, or are actively turning away from breastfeeding as a choice, because of the way they are feeling as a result of the operation.

Having a partner/birth companion present

Many studies have shown that women express greater satisfaction with birth, including caesarean section, when their partner or friend has been present for the delivery (see Chapter 11). The current study has demonstrated that the benefits to women of having a birth companion are immeasurable. Not only can they offer support and comfort at a personal level, they can act as advocate for the woman and fill in any 'missing pieces' about the birth.

> 'It was nice to know that my husband was there to see the birth and that I was able to talk to him right through the operation.'

'It was wonderful to be able to have my husband with me in theatre and to be talked through the whole thing – wouldn't have missed it for anything.'

These comments are from women who had their caesareans under regional anaesthesia. The benefits, therefore, to women having their caesareans under general anaesthetic are obvious. Their partner can support them and explain what happened during delivery, which will reduce the woman's feelings of having missed out on the birth. However, the results of the current study have demonstrated that it is precisely these women who are more likely to be denied the opportunity to have a friend or partner present and are thereby denied the benefits of this support.

In 1991/2 just over half the women in the sample had a partner with them during the operation. This was particularly the case for women having elective operations where two out of three women had their friend/partner present. However, less than half the women having emergency operations were accompanied during the operation. By 1996 almost two in three women (64.6 per cent) in the sample were reporting that their partners were present for the operation. But the difference between those having emergency and elective operations remained (54.0 per cent and 76.8 per cent respectively). Whether or not a partner or companion is allowed into the operating theatre is, more often than not, dependent on the preference of the doctor attending the birth. The findings of the current study are consistent with results from a survey of consultants' views on caesarean section which found that just under half of consultants said that friends/partners are invited into the theatre for caesarean births and a similar number said that they are 'sometimes' invited. Those consultants who answered that they sometimes invited the woman's friend/partner to be present for the operation were asked what the decision depended upon. Of those consultants who do place restrictions on patient support during the operation, the use of a spinal or epidural anaesthetic was by far the most common precondition. One consultant said:

'I always invite the husband if we are using an epidural but would not usually for general anaesthetic.'

Another said that the partner/companion would be invited to attend 'unless there were contra-indications such as a general anaesthetic'. Others were not specific about type of anaesthetic used but referred instead to whether the operation was emergency or elective. One doctor said he would allow the observer into the theatre 'if it was the woman's wish and it was not an emergency caesarean for fetal distress'. Another summed-up the feelings of many with two pre-conditions for the partner's attendance. These were that 'the caesarean was elective and under epidural' (Francome et al., 1993, pp. 136–37).

The results of the current study further demonstrate that although more partners are being allowed to be present for caesarean births (64.6 per cent in 1996 compared to 55.0 per cent in 1991/2), less women having emergency operations are accompanied. Furthermore, when looking at the type of anaesthetic used for the operation and partners' presence, it is clear that general anaesthetic acts as a bar to many partners with one in thirteen women who had general anaesthetic for their caesarean sections in the 1996 study being accompanied for the operation. This represented a dramatic drop in partners' presence for general anaesthetic operations over the five years of study as the 1991/2 data demonstrated that one in three caesarean-delivered women having general anaesthetic had their partner present for the operation. A small proportion of this anomaly will be accounted for by the fact that a slightly higher proportion of general anaesthetic caesareans were emergency operations in the 1996 sample because of the reduced use of general anaesthesia for elective caesareans. But this cannot account for the whole story. Potential methodological problems are discussed in Chapter 12 but are unlikely to account for the discrepancy totally. Personal correspondence with some of the Consultants in the sample suggest that there has been no change in practice regarding partners' presence at general anaesthetic caesareans. Clearly further research is required in this area.

The preferences of the consultant attending the birth have an impact on whether or not partners are permitted into the theatre during the birth. From the results of the current survey of women's experiences of caesarean section it is clear that women are very much aware of this fact. The women who did not have a companion or partner present for the birth were asked why not. The overwhelming majority of reasons given by women were to do with hospital/doctor policy regarding caesarean sections, particularly in relation to the administration of general anaesthetic. When asked why they did not have a partner or friend present for the birth the women said, for example: 'he had to go out when I had the general anaesthetic', 'he stayed until the general anaesthetic' and 'he didn't get into theatre during the operation'.

What emerged from the results of this study is that the majority of women would prefer to have their partner/companion with them during the birth and it is the organization of hospital services which is preventing this. If the main reason for not allowing partners into the operating theatre is because the operation is being performed under general anaesthetic, then surely this is another indication that women should be given epidural or spinal block anaesthetic for caesarean section wherever possible.

Therefore it appears that women who have caesareans do suffer despite their subjective perceptions of their experiences which suggest that they do not feel that they have suffered. The evidence produced by this study has clearly proven the first hypothesis that, to a certain extent at least, caesarean birth denies women the opportunity of having a satisfying experience of childbirth and increases their suffering.

Conflict in maternity services – revisited

In Chapter eight, I argued that there is a conflict in maternity services between lay and professional perceptions of childbirth. In this chapter I have suggested that the conflict between women and obstetricians has led to women suffering as a result of childbirth practice, namely caesarean section. Yet the results of the present research into women's experiences of caesarean birth have shown that, subjectively, women do not feel as though they suffer as a result of their treatment in hospital. I further suggested that this result may, in part, be due to a design fault in the survey whereby women were asked to complete questionnaires whilst still under the care of hospital staff which may have had an effect on the comments that they felt able to make. However, I believe that there are much more subtle forces at work here. Women say that they do not suffer as a result of caesarean section because they do not believe that they suffer. Evidence from the current research and other studies has demonstrated categorically that women having caesareans do suffer. The important question is: why do women not perceive that they suffer as a result of abdominal delivery?

The answer to this question is that women believe their operations to be necessary, life-saving procedures, without which they would not have achieved the birth of their babies. In situations where women are being told that a caesarean is in the best interest of their about-to-be-born babies, few would argue, object or complain. What is crucial here, is the relationship between women and their medical attendants.

Mavis Kirkham, in her research, observed that many women in labour frequently apologize for themselves, their appearance, their behaviour, their requests, their being there, even during routine care. The implication here is that women in labour see themselves as rather a nuisance, possibly not behaving well and certainly not having any automatic right to the attention of the medical practitioners (Kirkham, 1986). This could be one of the reasons why many women do not complain about interventionist techniques such as caesarean section, or feel that they have any right to question the superior knowledge of the obstetricians. Rather, women are more likely to feel grateful for the expertise, skill and authority offered to them and obliged to the doctors for their time, attention and trouble in helping them (the women) out of a difficult situation. The results of the current study support this.

> 'I lost a lot of blood and am only too grateful the Consultant and his team for successfully completing my operation.'

> 'I was overwhelmed with gratitude when they delivered our baby.'

> 'As soon as they said you will have to have a section, I became very upset and cried a lot, even though I thoroughly understood the circumstances and knew it was for the very best for my baby and me. But as soon as I came round and saw my husband with my beautiful son I was glad it was all over and glad I had a section.'

> 'It was unavoidable and in the best interests of the baby. Whilst it will take a while to recover it is comforting to know the baby is now safe and well.'

It appears that women in labour are encouraged to feel extremely grateful for the treatment and attention they are given by the highly trained professionals. Thus when women do not receive the care or information they would like, few protest. Although the respondents in the current study expressed a high level of satisfaction with the amount of information they received about their condition, it appears that even when women are not given enough information they tend to accept what little they have been given and adapt to make the best of the information, conditions and choices available to them. They do not express dissatisfaction when they do not receive the information they require (Shapiro et al., 1983). It is more common for women to react in a way that allows them to view the situation from a different angle, to explain the lack of information and choice in terms of inadequate facilities or staff shortages. This prevents women getting angry about their situation, hence they do not harbour grievances and are able to maintain good relationships with the health care professionals (Cartwright, 1979). Similarly, respondents in the present study would not say that they had suffered as a result of the caesarean operation. They were grateful that the procedure had been made available to them.

Many women would not question a doctor's authority, particularly when they are told that the treatment they are about to receive is the best interest of their soon-to-be-born baby. Furthermore, few women would be willing to take responsibility for their decisions when the impression they get from the medical practitioners is that they will 'wash their hands' of them if they do not comply with medical advice. It has been suggested that the authority of the medical professionals, and the language used by them, puts women in a vulnerable position in that they have to take the advice of the doctors or face the consequences of their decisions (Oakley and Richards, 1990).

With caesarean section, the fact that an operation is about to be performed suggests to women as patients that a medical decision has been taken on the basis of 'need' alone. Therefore women who may question the use of other interventions, such as induction, will accept caesarean section without resistance (Oakley and Richards, 1990).

It is not surprising therefore that women assume an apologetic role given the intrinsically inferior and vulnerable position they are in, first, because they are in labour, and secondly, because they are placed in hospital as a patient. Given the imbalance of power between women and doctors, it is questionable that even when women are adequately informed about their condition and treatment they are in a position to assert their wishes and preferences.

It has been suggested that the lack of research being carried out into the effects of caesarean section is the result of a shared view amongst patients and professionals that the operation is 'essential' and that there is little relevance in ascertaining the feelings of those who have undergone a 'lifesaving' procedure (Oakley, 1983). However, the results support the view that women see the caesarean operation as entirely necessary and are reluctant to question its use. Not only do women feel that they have not suffered as a result of the operation, they also express a great deal of satisfaction with the amount of information they receive about their condition, their babies' health and the treatment they have received. Further, the majority believe that they understand why their caesareans were necessary. What is even more surprising is that of the women who did not see their babies immediately after delivery, only one in three reported negative feelings such as 'sad/upset', 'worried' or 'anxious'. The majority expressed positive or neutral emotions such as 'pleased', 'fine' and 'resigned'. The lack of questioning or concern over the necessity for the operation and related procedures, such as routine separation between mother and child following the birth, among women having caesareans, points to the fact that the procedure is viewed as an essential medical intervention that would not be used unless completely necessary.

Unfortunately, women's faith in the medical profession may be misguided. The results of a survey of consultants' attitudes about caesarean section found that almost half the doctors in Britain say that caesarean rates are rising because of fear of litigation (Francome et al., 1993), thereby demonstrating that factors other than medical necessity are affecting decisions on whether or not to perform a caesarean. In Chapter Ten, I outlined the various non-medical determinants which affect caesarean section rates, including consultant preference, medical convenience and financial considerations. Such an anomaly between women's perceptions of the necessity of caesarean section and doctors' rationales for performing the operation highlight a clear conflict between the two.

Women's faith in the medical profession must, in some cases, be misplaced because they are often not given all the information they need to make informed choices. Women feel they are kept sufficiently informed because they believe what they are told. If they are not given information, it is because it is not necessary for them. Clearly doctors are not going to tell women that they need a caesarean in order to cover the obstetrician against litigation. When this occurs it represents an abuse of power by the medical profession who know that women are not in a position to question or contend their authority. Women do not know that decisions are being made about their bodies on the basis of anything other than medical need.

The results of the current study have demonstrated clearly that women do suffer as a result of caesarean section. Not only in terms of physical and emotional sequelae, but also in terms of the abuse of power by the medical profession in not giving women the appropriate information that they need to make informed decisions regarding their care. In the following chapter I discuss what can be done to overcome these problems and make recommendations on how maternity services can be improved to ensure a better outcome, not just for women, but also their babies, families and hospital staff, including obstetricians.

CHAPTER FOURTEEN

Conclusions and Recommendations

In Chapter 12, Hypothesis Two stated that maternity services can be improved with regard to caesarean section, to ensure a better outcome for women.

The research question was therefore: what can be done to improve the outcome for women of childbirth in general, and caesarean section in particular?

This chapter will answer the question by drawing together information detailed in earlier sections and making recommendations for the future practice of caesarean birth.

The evidence presented throughout the latter half of this book has shown that rates of caesarean section are higher than can be justified in terms of infant or maternal outcomes. What is more, women suffer as a result of the number of operations being performed. This chapter concludes the study with summaries of the main findings of the research together with recommendations on how maternity care relating to caesarean section can be improved to ensure a better outcome, not only for women, but also their children, their families and hospital staff.

Recommendation No. 1:
A more selective use of caesarean section

Rates of caesarean section have been rising in all countries for which data are available. The latest calculation puts the caesarean rate in Britain at over 15 per cent (Francome, 1994). Although the rates for some countries appear to be stabilizing, there is no evidence to suggest that a caesarean rate above six per cent can be justified (Francome and Huntingford, 1980).

High caesarean section rates cannot be justified in terms of reductions in perinatal and neonatal mortality and have led to iatrogenic morbidity in babies born by section. Effects on women having caesareans have been even more severe and include increased risk of fatality. The results of the current study have shown that women who have caesarean deliveries report increased pain, immobility and lengthy recovery periods. They experience disappointment at not being able (or allowed) to give birth naturally. They feel shock, anger and increased psychological distress. They miss out on participating in the delivery of their babies and often miss the first minutes following the birth. Many caesarean mothers are routinely separated from their babies after delivery or feel too ill to care for their infants and therefore experience deleterious effects on bonding and breastfeeding as a result of giving birth by caesarean. What this means is that not only are women being denied positive experiences of childbirth but caesarean section may actually have long-term deleterious effects on the mother-child relationship and therefore the subsequent development of caesarean children.

The difference in caesarean rates between countries, regions, hospitals and individual consultants cannot be accounted for in terms of biological or medical differences in the populations of women served, and point to differences in practice rather than medical need. Some differences in caesarean rates rest upon extraneous variables including: socio-economic factors; consultant's preference; outdated practices, such as 'repeat caesareans'; hospital/doctor convenience; staff shortages; increased use of technology, especially electronic fetal monitoring; and the fear of litigation.

The ethical considerations associated with caesarean birth are not specific to this procedure but follow established patterns governing the relationship between health care providers and their patients. In 1981 the NIH Consensus Development Statement on Caesarean Section in the United States specified that the ethical guidelines should be:

> 'A commitment to giving patients' interests priority over their own and acknowledging the right of patients to make informed decisions regarding their own bodies.' (p. 23)

It is astonishing to see that such a statement still needs to be enforced. Caesarean sections continue to be performed for reasons other than medical necessity. Fear of litigation and financial factors being major considerations, demonstrating that doctors' interests are given priority over those of the patient.

Most of the extraneous factors can be overcome by education, peer pressure and/or social policy. Variables relating to doctor/hospital policy and preference will only change as a result of public and professional pressure highlighting the negative side-effects of caesarean birth and the lack of evidence to support higher rates of surgical intervention. There is some indication that this is beginning to happen with reduction in the number of operations performed for indications such as previous caesareans (Paterson and Saunders, 1991; Francome et al., 1993) (See Chapter 12).

The problem of caesareans being performed because of staff shortages and over-reliance on more junior doctors will not be solved until money is made available to staff labour wards appropriately and not over-stretching existing personnel. Such variables are intrinsically linked to governmental and Hospital Trust policies and priorities. Unfortunately, in times of economic recession, solutions which appear to require increased spending, for example on staffing and training, are not favourably received. Yet caesareans are more expensive than vaginal deliveries. Calculations have demonstrated that a reduction of only one per cent in the caesarean section rate in Britain would save the health service £7,000,000 a year (Savage and Francome, 1993).

In times of scarce resourcing for health services, it must surely be inappropriate to channel money into interventionist techniques, such as the caesarean section, which may be of questionable value.

There is a wealth of evidence to suggest that VBAC is a safe and preferable alternative to repeat caesareans for most women. Some change in medical attitude, and thus practice, is also evident but there is still some reluctance to change on the part of many obstetricians. Even when convinced of the intellectual rationale that VBAC is safe, it appears that situational pressures, including anxiety over legal liability, the inconvenience of lengthy labours, peer pressure and general resistance to change, predispose obstetricians to retain familiar, yet outdated, patterns of behaviour. Thus doctors not only need to be made aware of the feasibility and safety of VBAC, but also need encouragement to change their practice, coupled with support against litigation, if they are to assist women to attempt VBAC, thereby reducing the number of unnecessary repeat caesareans.

However, there is evidence to suggest that some women prefer elective caesarean sections to the potential discomfort of a trial of labour, especially after a previous experience of prolonged labour and eventual caesarean. The results of the current research and evidence from previous studies demonstrate that fear of failed trial of labour and the convenience of a scheduled delivery, coupled with negative attitudes from obstetricians towards a trial of labour, all contribute to women's choice of elective caesarean section. Yet in hospitals where VBAC is encouraged, two thirds of eligible women choose trial of labour and the majority succeed in achieving vaginal birth (Shepperd McClain, 1990). What this points to is that women need to be made aware of the feasibility and success of VBAC if they are to make informed choices.

Where population differences are evident in caesarean section rates they tend to be closely related to social class. Such social class differentials are usually associated with the difference between public and private health care with the private sector having the highest section rates. This is the case for all countries where a two-tier system of health care operates including Britain, Italy, the United States and Brazil.

The high rate of caesareans among women in the higher socio-economic groups is also associated with another extraneous, or non-medical variable which, in turn, increases the rate still further. It is fear of litigation. It used to be the case that only the more affluent sectors of the population would sue the medical profession in the event of a catastrophe occurring during treatment. This is therefore, in part, responsible for the high caesarean rate among this group. Yet with increasing awareness among the general population (and possibly the Patient's Charter), coupled with changes in procedures for claiming legal aid instituted in 1990, legal action following problems at birth have nearly doubled (Macnair, 1992). Seventy per cent of the obstetric consultants in a small-scale British study cited fear of litigation as a reason for the rising caesarean rate (Francome, 1994). What is more, fear of litigation increases stress and anxiety levels among doctors and is responsible for turning large numbers of junior doctors away from obstetrics as a career and the early retirement of older practitioners (Macnair, 1992). This clearly exacerbates the problem of staff shortages which, in turn, leads to more caesareans.

There are two main ways of overcoming the problem of defensive medicine. First the introduction of no-fault compensation for birth injuries, thereby acknowledging that parents of children damaged at birth need support regardless of allocation of blame. At the same time a procedure of close monitoring of standards of medical practice, coupled with litigation if the standard of medical treatment falls below an acceptable level, should ensure that doctors are not punished for decisions made in good faith and women receive treatment commensurate with their condition.

Secondly, continuity of care for women during pregnancy and labour will enable relationships to be built between the two. It is when these relationships are absent, when women see a range of different professionals each time they visit the hospital, that mistrust and resentment can develop. The number of caesareans being performed because of fear of litigation can, therefore, be reduced if women are given continuity of care and enabled to build relationships with the health care professionals based on mutual trust. This reduces the risk of women blaming the midwife or doctor in the event of something going wrong with the birth.

There is some evidence to suggest that this message is now being heard by government agencies. The report of the expert maternity group 'Changing Childbirth' recommended both continuity of maternity care and an improvement in communication between the providers and recipients of care (Expert Maternity Group, 1993). However, rather than reducing the number of caesareans, it has been suggested that this document has actually lead to an increase in the section rate (Savage, in Francome, 1994). It appears that giving women choice in maternity services means that more women request caesarean section. The results of the current research certainly support this with the number of women requesting the operation rising from 13.2 per cent in 1991/2 to 21.3 per cent in 1996. The problem here is that the 'Changing Childbirth' document recommends giving women informed choice. The question is whether women opting for caesarean section are actually making informed decisions. The number of women reporting 'shock' and 'frustration' in the current study would suggest that women are not adequately prepared. It may therefore be that when women 'choose' a caesarean birth they do so on preconceived ideas and misconceptions about this mode of delivery.

Obviously there will always be situations where a caesarean is necessary and there will always be women who need surgical interventions to enable them to deliver their babies. But the evidence suggesting that neonatal and perinatal outcomes are not improved by caesarean section rates above six per cent and the wealth of evidence highlighting the negative sequelae of caesarean birth for women, their babies and the relationship between the two, point to the fact that it is clearly unacceptable to carry out caesarean section for any other reason than medical need. Every caesarean should be a necessary caesarean.

Recommendation No. 2:
Less use of emergency caesareans

Evidence from this study has demonstrated that while some important improvements in the experiences of women having emergency caesarean operations are apparent, on the whole women who have emergency caesareans have less positive perceptions of the delivery than women who have elective caesarean deliveries and report significantly more distress regarding the physical sensations associated with the birth. The current study found that women who have emergency operations report negative post-operative feelings, such as 'tiredness' and 'weakness', more than women who have elective caesareans. Women who have elective caesareans report positive post-operative feelings, such as 'happiness', more than women who have emergency sections.

Evidence demonstrates that early and continued contact between mother and child is important for the development of the relationship between the two. Adding to the problems of emergency caesarean birth is the fact that women are often separated from their babies following delivery as some babies may be taken into intensive care units as a matter of routine. Respondents in the current study also reported that their physical state post-surgery and general feelings of being unwell affect their ability to care for their infants and may have an impact on bonding. Almost three times as many women delivered by emergency caesarean said that this was the case, compared to those who had elective operations. Women who have had emergency caesareans may therefore experience adverse effects on their relationships with their children. In other words, their ability to bond appropriately with their children may be put in jeopardy because of emergency caesarean operations.

The increased negative sequelae experienced by women having emergency caesareans can be explained in terms of lack of preparation for, and expectation of abdominal delivery. From the results of the present research, it is clear that lack of mental and physical preparation amongst emergency caesarean patients leads to increased psychological and physical morbidity. This evidence suggests that the unplanned or emergency caesarean delivery may have more influence on the woman's experience of birth than the caesarean delivery per se.

When the caesarean is elective, the woman has time to acquire the knowledge and information she will need to deal appropriately with the operation. She will have time to read about caesarean birth and to discuss any queries with health professionals which should enable her to come to terms with what is about to happen and thereby avoid the feelings of complete disappointment that many emergency caesarean patients feel. The need for women to be better prepared for the possibility of caesarean birth at the antenatal stage is addressed in 'Recommendation No. 4'. But, what this evidence points to is the need for caesareans, when medically indicated, to be elective in all possible cases, thereby enabling the woman to familiarize herself with the procedures and after-effects of caesarean birth in order to avoid some of the negative repercussions that many women currently suffer.

Results of the current research have shown that over half the caesareans in both samples were emergency operations. The latest data showed that three quarters (75.2 per cent) of the emergency operations were performed because labour was taking a long time (dystocia) and/or the baby was distressed (fetal distress). Yet both of these diagnostic categories envelope many conditions and, as such, lend themselves to individual interpretation. Further, they have the potential for over-use in situations where medical staff are unclear of how to proceed or are unwilling to proceed with a labour that they perceive to be 'difficult'. There are two main problems associated with the use of vague diagnostic categories. The first is that doctors and midwives become deskilled in the management of labours that, for whatever reason, are not perceived to be 'normal', and secondly, the medical labels 'dystocia' and 'fetal distress' given as rationale for caesarean operations imply to women that decisions have been made on the basis of medical need alone. Thus women are unlikely to question such medical decisions and are thereby disempowered in the delivery process as they are not able to make informed choices about their care.

The increasing use of technology to manage labour and the fact that the use of one intervention tends to lead to a whole sequence of interventions means that medical students, doctors and midwives in training do not see as many normal labours as they need to in order to understand the individual pattern of an average range of women in labour (Savage, 1986). The staffing of labour wards by registrars and other relatively junior staff tends to lead to an increase in the use of emergency caesarean operations because the doctors do not have the skill or experience to proceed with labours which do not fit in with the expected average time scales for labour.

The answer to this problem is, first, to increase education and understanding about the whole spectrum of differences in labour rather than relying on estimates of an average range of women in labour. Secondly, to revive obstetric skills which appear to have been lost over time such as external version, instead of resorting to caesarean section in all cases other than vertex presentation. Finally, a solution to this problem would be to have labours managed by midwives who are often more experienced in the range of different labours and are less likely than obstetricians to resort to interventionist techniques to aid delivery. In this way, the majority of women who do not need medical or surgical interventions will not be subjected to them, and the skills and expertise of the obstetricians will be utilized appropriately for the minority of women who need them.

What this means is that women will not be subjected to emergency caesarean sections because their labours do not fit into an average calculation of women in labour, or because medical staff attending the labour do not have experience of dealing with a full range of different deliveries. Less emergency caesareans, with the accompanying negative sequelae, will mean more positive experiences of childbirth for women.

Recommendation No. 3:
The use of regional anaesthetic in all possible cases of caesarean section

It is clear that women who have emergency caesarean operations have less positive experiences than those who have elective operations. What is also clear is that the negative effects of emergency caesareans are compounded by the use of general anaesthesia. This means that a substantial proportion of caesarean patients are being denied a satisfactory experience of childbirth. Caesarean delivered women who have had regional anaesthesia tend to report more positive experiences of birth than those who have their operations under regional anaesthesia.

The use of general anaesthesia for caesarean section has reduced over the period of study from 58.0 per cent of caesareans in the 1991/2 study to 32.5 per cent in the 1996 survey. This is an encouraging trend. However 65.0 per cent of caesarean operation performed with women under general anaesthetic are emergency sections. Thus the use of general anaesthetic coupled with emergency operations combine to compound negative experiences of caesarean section in many cases.

Caesarean-delivered women who have had regional anaesthesia tend to report more positive experiences of birth than those who have their operations under general anaesthetic. The results of the current study have shown that women who remain conscious for their caesarean operations feel as though they have taken part in the delivery of their babies. It appears that being awake for the birth is analogous to having participated for many women. Other studies have demonstrated that regional anaesthesia allows women to retain a sense of control over what is happening and therefore increases their satisfaction with the birth process (Sargent and Stark, 1987).

The use of regional anaesthesia for caesarean section also makes it easier for women in the early postnatal period as they are not recovering from the effects of general anaesthetic and are therefore more free to respond to their babies' needs. The majority of women in the current study who reported that they did not see their baby immediately after the delivery said that this was because they were waiting for the effects of the general anaesthetic to wear off.

Partners or birth companions are frequently permitted to be present for caesarean births when regional anaesthesia is being used. The current study demonstrated that partners are increasingly excluded when general anaesthetic is administered. The proportion of women having general anaesthetic for their caesareans and having a partner present for the delivery has reduced over the five year period of study from 33.7 per cent among the 1991/2 sample to 7.6 per cent in 1996. The results of a survey of consultants' views on caesarean section confirmed that the use of general anaesthesia is cited by doctors as a contra-indication for allowing partners into the operating theatre (Francome et al., 1993). Yet women report greater satisfaction with caesarean delivery when they have been able to share it with their partner or birth companion. It may be that this is deemed to be unimportant for women having general anaesthesia as, after all, they are asleep during the birth. But one of the benefits of having a partner present during delivery is that they can share their recollections of the birth and fill in any missing pieces. The benefits to women having general anaesthesia are therefore obvious.

Evidence from other studies has also shown that the negative effects of the use of general anaesthesia for caesarean operations are that it increases post-operative morbidity (Morgan et al., 1984; Lelong and Kaminski, 1987; Oakley and Richards, 1990), and not least of all, general anaesthesia is associated with increased rates of maternal mortality (DoH, 1991 and 1994).

Although it was not within the remit of the present study to examine the long-term effects of caesarean birth, work by other researchers has demonstrated a link between the use of general anaesthesia and detrimental effects on the mother-baby relationship (Gottlieb and Barratt, 1986).

What is surprising is that a significant proportion (24.5 per cent) of women who had elective operations in the 1996 survey also had general anaesthesia. Yet the reasons that may be given for the use of general anaesthesia in emergency situations, such as the presence of fetal distress or dystocia, are less likely to apply in an elective caesarean situation. It appears, therefore, that general anaesthesia is being used for elective operations for other reasons. It may be that women are reluctant to be awake for major surgery. If this is the case, it reflects a lack of information and hence knowledge among childbearing women about the benefits of being awake for caesarean birth. It may also be a reflection of hospital or consultant policy which dictates that women are under general anaesthesia for caesarean operations.

Of course one of the most important outcomes of any pregnancy is the birth of a healthy baby. Yet for women, success in childbirth may also mean more in terms of a personally satisfying experience, leading to a sense of accomplishment and not to a sense of failure and loss of control. What this means is that the over-use of general anaesthesia for caesarean birth is denying women a satisfactory experience of childbirth and a fulfilling start to motherhood. It is clear therefore that the needs of women may not always be taken into account when decisions are made about anaesthesia for caesarean operations.

The answer, and therefore the recommendation of this study, is that the experience of women who have to undergo caesarean section could be improved if they are awake for the operation. Thus regional anaesthesia should be used for caesarean section in all possible cases.

Recommendation No. 4:
Women should be fully informed at all stages of treatment

The results of the current study have shown that women who are better prepared for caesarean birth have a more rewarding experience overall. Thus, for example, women who have had previous caesareans tend to report greater satisfaction with their treatment before the operation, during it and post-operatively. There are two main reasons for this. First, women having second or third caesareans are more likely to have elective operations, thus they do not expect a vaginal birth and are not subsequently disappointed that this has been denied. A related point is that women are more often given epidural or spinal anaesthetic for elective operations and it has been demonstrated through the current research that women who are awake for the birth of their babies feel much better about the caesarean than those who are given general anaesthetic. Secondly, women having subsequent operations are better prepared mentally for all that caesarean birth entails. They are aware of the after-effects of the operation, they know that it will be painful, they do not expect to be up and about doing everything for their newborn. What this points to is the need for women to be appropriately prepared during their pregnancy for the possibility of caesarean birth.

One respondent in the current study, interviewed some time after her emergency caesarean, said about the operation:

'Ten months on, it is still frequently on my mind. I crave for answers to questions that I know will probably never be answered, such as: What if I had gone another hour, would it have made a difference? What if I had been under a different Consultant? When I am ready to have my next child, I will do everything in my power to avoid repeating the experience as, although physically I healed very quickly, mentally, the wound is still as fresh as the day it was made.'

One of the most startling observations to come out of this research is the fact that most women are completely unprepared for operative delivery. Although caesarean birth is currently mentioned at antenatal classes, it must be noted that not all women attend these classes, and the philosophy 'it'll never happen to me' comes into play in this situation, particularly when the pregnancy has been unproblematic.

It also points to the fact that there is a lack of understanding generally about caesarean birth. Women who have not experienced it often see it as a 'soft' option and do not realize the pain, discomfort, lack of mobility and lengthy recovery that it entails. What this indicates is that all pregnant women need to have full knowledge of caesarean section, whether they are deemed to be 'at risk' in terms of possibly needing a section or not. Similarly, medical staff need to be sensitive to the post-operative needs and feelings of women who have had caesareans, as they will not always be able to deal with their newborns as well as they had expected to and this can cause stress and depression.

From the comments made by the women in the present study it is clear to see that many women experience very mixed feelings about the operation. Obviously they are thankful that it is available and understand the necessity of it in certain circumstances. Yet because the majority of women are incapacitated by the surgery they are unable to fulfill what they see as their obligations to their newborn babies. This will inevitably lead to conflict for the women concerned.

It appears that, on the whole, women feel as though they are kept informed about their condition and that of their baby, about the treatment they are given and about the reasons for the operation. However, information is lacking in terms of the procedure for caesarean section and the effects on women post-operatively. It is clear from the results of the current research that women require more information about caesareans. This includes what to expect both during and after the procedure and the implications of being awake or asleep for the operation. All antenatal classes should incorporate this information as well as caesarean statistics. Thus women might realize that the experience is not so rare and that there are choices they can make both to reduce the risk of a caesarean occurring and to make the experience, if it happens to them, as well as its aftermath, as positive as possible. If women are to make informed decisions about what happens to them in hospital and to be empowered to take a full and rewarding part in the birth of their children, they need to realize that caesarean birth is a very real possibility for many, and they need appropriate information in order to reduce feelings of shock, disappointment and resentment.

Evidence discussed in Chapter eight highlighted the problem of communication between health professionals and pregnant women as recipients of health care. One bar to communication was identified as confusion over who should take responsibility for informing women. The 'Changing Childbirth' document was cited as a positive move towards enabling women to make informed decisions about their care through the imparting of appropriate information from a professional that the woman knows and has been able to develop a relationship with through continuity of care. Clearly this has worked to a degree. Women in the current study certainly reported that they felt adequately informed. However, evidence suggests that not only is there room for improvement in the communication between women and their attendants during childbirth, but also that some information given to women by their attendants in hospital is, at best inadequate, and at worst, untruthful. Inconsistencies in the results of the current research compared with findings from a survey of consultants' views on caesarean section illustrate this. Almost three quarters (70.0 per cent) of the doctors gave 'fear of litigation' as a reason for the increase in caesarean section rates (Francome et al., 1993), yet women are told that their caesareans are necessary for reasons of dystocia or fetal distress. Similarly, whilst evidence from previous research suggests that caesareans are performed for the convenience of medical staff, women are given medical rationale for their operations. Clearly women are not being given the correct information and, as such, are disempowered in childbirth. Without adequate information women are not able to make informed choices.

Peter Huntingford, a consultant obstetrician who has spoken in favour of women's right to control childbirth said in 1985:

> 'In my opinion, the practice of obstetrics for defensive reasons is totally unjustified and misguided. If doctors were not so arrogant and were more truthful, they would not need to practise in this way. All they have to do is to reveal their own weaknesses and lack of knowledge. For most doctors, the most truthful response they could give in many cases would be: "I don't know what the cause is or what is the best course of action". Doctors would not need to practise defensively if they were willing to say: "This is the situation as I see it: we could do this or that, but I am not really sure what is best. Under these circumstances, what would you prefer me to do?" In my experience, by sharing responsibility like this I am more likely to make the best decision and furthermore (although this is a secondary consideration), I am less likely to be blamed when the outcome is tragedy. Being truthful and sharing responsibility is not opting out. It does not absolve us from responsibility. It is the more difficult course to follow, since it requires more time, more emotional involvement and more consideration of the wishes of others rather than of our own.' (pp. 6–7)

In the same year, the World Health Organization (WHO) published a statement on the use of technology in childbirth which recommended that:

> 'Technology assessment should involve all those using the technology, epidemiologists, social scientists, health authorities and the women on whom the technology is used.' (p. 437)

165

What is most unfortunate is the fact that over a decade since the WHO's recommendations on the use of technology in childbirth were published, women are still not being empowered to take a full and meaningful role in the delivery of their children.

Clearly Huntingford's sentiments echo the recommendations of the WHO statement. His suggested solution is that in order to give the patients needs and wishes priority over those of the medical practitioners, doctors need to give more time and be prepared to make an emotional investment in their relationships with their patients. Further, this requires them to be more honest, particularly when the required course of action is not clear-cut. To acknowledge this uncertainty and to share it with the patient, who, after all, has the right to know.

The recommendation of this study, therefore, is a complete reorganization of the doctor-patient relationship. For doctors, this means giving up some of their power and authority. Consultants and hospital staff need more information too. They need to know about caesarean section rates, about the benefits and hazards of performing the operation and, more specifically, they need to be made aware of the effect that abdominal delivery has on women and their babies in the short and long term. What is also clear is that doctors need more information in relation to the number of caesareans being carried out by their hospital in general, and about their individual practise in particular, such audit and monitoring have been shown to reduce caesarean section rates.

Not only is it the case that the medical professions need to be encouraged to impart information to women to empower them to participate in decision-making and to enable them to feel as though they have taken a full and meaningful role in the birth of their babies, but health practitioners need to ensure that the information given to women is accurate and imparted at a level that is accessible to the women concerned. Only then will a 'successful' outcome be achieved by women as well as doctors.

For women, the reorganization of the doctor/patient relationship means taking control over their bodies. In 1979, Ann Cartwright stated:

> 'The women's movement may have raised expectations and heightened awareness among some women, but it has a long way to go in giving women the confidence and ability to challenge and change services rather than passively to accept them.' (pp. 163–64)

Cartwright's answer to this problem is that women should be encouraged to first, ask more questions rather than waiting and hoping to find out what they want to know, to not allow themselves to be 'fobbed off' with answers that do not give them the information they require, and to overcome their reluctance to expose their ignorance and uncertainties. Secondly, to make their own wishes and preferences known and to demand to know why their stated preferences are ignored. Finally, women should be encouraged to insist on being involved in important decisions that are made about them.

However, it appears that almost 20 years on we still have a long way to go. If women are to be empowered in this way it would necessarily involve a complete reorganization of the relationship between pregnant women and medical professionals whereby doctors relinquish some of their control. Only then will the patient be able to take an active role in decision-making about her body and her treatment, she will be empowered to make an informed choice rather than relying totally on the decision of the medical practitioners. Studies have demonstrated that women do want to be informed about issues relating to caesarean birth including the reasons and rationale behind performing the operation and the medical and surgical complications associated with caesarean delivery. Women need this information in order to take part in decisions that are made about them and to participate as fully as possible in the delivery of their babies. However, the results of the present study suggest that, in the hospital situation, women are prepared to rely totally on the judgement of the doctors and in some respects, expect to be told what is happening and what will happen to them. Therefore it is not only the doctors who need to be re-socialized into a new way of thinking and relating to their patients. Women too need to be made aware of their rights, that their own knowledge and feelings about childbirth are valuable, and more importantly, that the doctor does not always know best.

Glossary

abdominal birth   Delivery of the baby via the abdomen, i.e. caesarean section, rather than the usual route along the vagina.

bi-cornuate uterus   The uterus is heart-shaped with two sections at the top end. This condition can cause difficulties during labour and may therefore indicate that a caesarean section is required.

cephalopelvic disproportion   A condition in pregnancy where there is disproportion between the size of the baby and the size of the pelvic opening. Either the pelvis is too small for the baby or the baby too big for the pelvis. It basically means that the baby cannot pass through the pelvic gap.

craniotomy   The perforation, breaking or crushing of the fetal skull in order to extract the infant (in pieces) through the vaginal canal.

elective (caesarean)   A caesarean performed before the onset of labour, usually pre-planned because of a foreseen condition such as the small size of the pelvis.

embriotomy   A procedure whereby the infant is mutilated in utero and extracted in pieces. Where the head is the part of the infant presenting, the process is referred to as craniotomy.

epidural anaesthesia   A form of local (regional) anaesthesia used to numb the abdomen for routine pain relief during labour and total pain relief during caesarean. The woman is awake for the operation when this type of anaesthesia is used.

emergency (caesarean)   A caesarean performed once labour has begun, not necessarily because of an 'emergency' in the conventional sense, but usually because of an unforeseen event or condition arising during labour. The unplanned nature of these operations usually means that normal preparatory measures for major surgery, such as a fasting period, are not observed.

external cephalic version	A procedure whereby an obstetrician or midwife attempts to move the infant in the uterus into a more favourable position for delivery by exerting external pressure on the woman's abdomen.
general anaesthesia	A combination of drugs used to anaesthetise the whole of the body by producing a state of unconsciousness.
infant mortality	Statistical measure of the number of deaths of infants during or just after birth, or within the first year of life.
litigation	The bringing of a lawsuit against a person. With reference to caesarean section 'fear of litigation' is used to describe the rationale for actions of obstetricians when operations are performed because the practitioner is afraid of being sued in the event of an unsuccessful outcome of childbirth.
medical ethos	The collection of attitudes, character, disposition and nature of the medical profession.
medical model	The shape or form of the group of attitudes which dominate the medical profession. The term is used particularly with reference to viewing illness as an isolated incident affecting a particular part of the body which can be treated in order to return the organism to as normal a state as possible, rather than taking into consideration social and environmental variables which affect health. In terms of obstetrics the medical model is associated with a view of pregnancy and childbirth as an illness requiring medical attention and, more often than not, treatment.
medical variables	Medical indications for caesarean section, that is, those medically defined conditions of the woman or the infant that are used to indicate the necessity of a caesarean operation. Such variables may be 'absolute' or 'relative'. Absolute medical variables are those conditions and situations where the only safe option for either the mother or the baby, or both, is to have a caesarean, e.g. disproportion between the size of the woman's pelvis and the size of the baby. Relative indications are more loosely defined conditions which may or may not require a caesarean such as dystocia and fetal distress.
neonatal	During the first month of life.

non-medical variables   Variables affecting the number of caesareans being performed but not based on an assessment of medical necessity. Such variables include consultants preference, fear of litigation and economic or staffing considerations.

objective response   For the purpose of this study, this term has been used to refer to an assessment of women's reactions to caesarean section, particularly in relation to their suffering, based on their responses to questions about the amount of pain they experienced, separation from their babies, support during delivery etc.

oblique presentation   The baby is lying diagonally across the womb during the time leading up to the birth.

pain   The concept of pain used in this study refers to women's subjective perception of the amount of physical pain they experienced as a result of the caesarean operation. However, it is suggested in this work that women's experience of pain may be affected by psycho-social considerations, such as not being adequately prepared for caesarean birth and expecting the operation to be relatively pain-free as compared to vaginal delivery.

perinatal   During the period from the twenty-fourth week of pregnancy to seven days after birth.

perinatal mortality rate   The rate (usually expressed per 1,000) of babies dying between the twenty-fourth week of pregnancy and seven days after birth.

placenta praevia   The placenta is situated in the lower part of the uterus. A caesarean section will be necessary if the placenta is covering the cervix and therefore preventing the baby's progress into the vagina.

power   The ability/capacity to influence the behaviour of others, either directly, for example, by being in a position to tell others what is best for them, or indirectly by having influence over policies and services provided for others.

primigravidae   Women giving birth for the first time.

spinal block   A form of local (regional) anaesthesia whereby an injection is given into the cerebrospinal fluid to numb the abdomen for a caesarean. The woman is awake during the operation when this type of anaesthetic is used.

subjective response   The personal response of women taking part in the survey based on their own perceptions of their experiences.

ventral conception   A pregnancy where the fetus grows outside of the womb.

References

Abitbol, M.M., Castillo, I., Taylor, U.B., Rochelson, B.L., Shoys, S., Monheit, A.G. (1993). 'Vaginal birth after cesarean section: the patient's point of view'. *American Family Physician*, 47(1), pp. 129–34.

Adashek, J.A., Peaceman, A.M., Lopez-Zeno, J.A., Minogue, J.P., Socol, M.L. (1993). 'Factors contributing to the increased cesarean birth rate in older parturient women'. *American Journal of Obstetrics and Gynecology*, 169(4), pp. 936–40.

Affonso, D., Stichler, J. (1980). 'Cesarean birth: Women's reactions'. *American Journal of Nursing*, March, pp. 468–70.

Albers, L.L., Savitz, D.A. (1991). 'Hospital setting for birth and use of medical procedures in low-risk women'. *Journal of Nurse Midwifery*, 36(6), pp. 327–33.

Allison, J. (1987). 'Highlights from the history of caesarean'. *Midwife, Health Visitor and Community Nurse*, 23(12), pp. 546–47.

Arthure et al. (1975). *Report on Confidential Inquiries into Maternal Deaths in England and Wales in 1970–72*. Reports of the Health Society, Subject No. 11, London: HMSO.

Axten, S. (1995). 'Is active management always necessary?'. *Modern Midwife*, 5(5), pp. 18–20.

Baliva, R., Serpieri, A. (1886). *The Lancet*, 5, 890 and 994.

Barlow, J. (1822). *Essays on Surgery and Midwifery*. London: Baldwin, Craddock and Joy.

Baruffi, G., Strobino, D.M., Paine, L.L. (1990). 'Investigation of institutional differences in primary cesarean birth rates'. *Journal of Nurse Midwifery*, 35(5), pp. 274–81.

Baudelocque, M. (1801). *Two Memoirs on the Cesarean Operation*. Translated from the French by John Hull, Manchester: Sowler and Russell.

Beal, J.A. (1993). 'Commentary on effects of information on adaptation to cesarean birth'. *Nursing Scan in Research*, 6(4), p. 5.

Bell, G. (1916). 'Caesarean section in a pitman's cottage'. *British Medical Journal*, 1, pp. 195–96.

Bertollini, R., DiLallo, D., Spadea, T., Perucci, C. (1992) 'Cesarean section rates in Italy by hospital payment mode: An analysis based on birth certificates'. *American Journal of Public Health*, 82, pp. 257–61.

Bewley, S., Robson, S.C., Smith, M., Glover, A., Spencer, J.A. (1993). 'The introduction of external cephalic version at term into routine clinical practice'. *European Journal of Obstetrics, Gynecology and Reproductive Biology*, 52(2), pp. 89–93.

Bishop, W.J. (1960). *The Early History of Surgery*. London: Robert Hale Ltd.

Blacker, G. (1921). 'The limitations of caesarean section'. *The Journal of Obstetrics and Gynaecology of the British Empire*, Index to Volume 28, pp. 447–62.

Bowers, S.K., MacDonald, I.T.M., Shapiro, E.D. (1982). 'Prevention of iatrogenic neonatal respiratory distress syndrome: elective repeat cesarean section and spontaneous labor'. *American Journal of Obstetrics and Gynaecology*, 143, pp. 186–89.

Boyd, C., Francome, C. (1986). *One Birth in Nine*. London: Maternity Alliance.

Boylan, P., Frankowski, R., Rountree, R., Selwyn, B., Parrish, K. (1991). 'Effect of active management of labor on the incidence of cesarean section for dystocia in nulliparas'. *American Journal of Perinatology*, 8(6), pp. 373–79.

Bradley, C.F. (1983). 'Psychological consequences of intervention in the birth process'. *Canadian Journal of Behavioural Science*, 15(4), pp. 422–38.

Brahams, D. (1988). 'A visit to the USA - part I'. *New Law Journal*, 138, pp. 361–63.

Bright Bannister, J. (1935). *British Medical Journal*, I, pp. 684–85.

Brith, K., Larsen, T., Torgersen, S. (1992). 'A longitudinal study of women in childbirth and their four-year-old children'. *Journal of Reproductive and Infant Psychology*, 10(3), pp. 177–82.

British Medical Journal (1922). 'Editorial'. I, pp. 277–78.

British Medical Journal (1936). 'Report of the meeting of the north of england obstetrical and gynaecological society'. 27 November, 2, pp. 1279–80.

Browne, A. (1994). 'Are midwives ready for the proposals for change?'. *Nursing Times*, 90(47), p. 37.

Burt, R.D., Vaughn, T.L., Daling, J.R. (1988). 'Evaluating the risks of caesarean section: low Apgar score in repeat cesarean section and vaginal deliveries'. *American Journal of Public Health*, 78, pp. 1312–14.

Butler, N.R., Bonham, D.G. (1963). *Perinatal Mortality*. London and Edinburgh: Livingstone.

Chamberlain, R., Chamberlain, G. (1975). *British Births*. London: Heinemann Medical Books.

Caffo, E., Guaraldi, G.P., Magnani, G., Tassi, R. (1982). 'Prevention of child abuse and neglect through early diagnosis of serious disturbances in the mother-child relationship in Italy'. *Child Abuse and Neglect*, 6, p. 453.

Cain, R.L. et al. (1984). 'Effects of father's presence or absence during a cesarean delivery'. *Birth*, 11, pp. 10–15.

Calhoun, B.C., Edgeworth, D., Brehm, W. (1995). 'External cephalic version at a military teaching hospital: predictors of success'. *Australian and New Zealand Journal of Obstetrics and Gynaecology*, 35(3), pp. 277–79.

Cameron, M. (1892). *British Medical Journal*. 3, p. 594.

Cappa, F., D'Alfonso, A., Di Luzio, F., Zaurito, V., Di Stefano, L. (1991). 'Indications and contra-indications for normal labor in patients who previously underwent cesarean section'. *Minerva Ginecologica*, 43(1–2), pp. 7–13.

Cardale, P. (1994) 'Changing role for midwives'. *Nursing Times*, 90(28), p. 60.

Cartwright, A. (1979). *The Dignity of Labour? A Study of Childbearing and Induction*. London: Tavistock.

C/SEC (1987). *Cesareans/Support Education and Concern Newsletter*. 13(3).

Chalmers, I., Richards, M. (1977). 'Intervention and causal inference in obstetric practice'. In: Chard, T., Richards, M. (Eds). *Benefits and Hazards of The New Obstetrics*. London: William Heinemann Medical Books.

Chamberlain, G. (1993). 'What is the correct caesarean section rate?'. *British Journal of Obstetrics and Gynaecology*, 100(5), pp. 403–04.

Clarke, R. (1994). 'Normal services will be resumed?'. *Modern Midwife*, 4(12), pp. 36–37.

Cohen, M., Carson, B.S. (1985). 'Respiratory morbidity benefit of awaiting onset of labour after elective cesarean section'. *Obstetrics and Gynaecology*, 65, pp. 818–24.

Cohen, N.W. (1977). 'Minimising emotional sequele of caesarean childbirth'. *Birth*, 4, pp. 114–19.

Cohnklin, M.M. (1977). 'Discussion groups as preparation for Cesarean section'. *Journal of Obstetrics, Gynaecology and Neonatal Nursing*, 6(4), pp. 52–54.

Comerio, D., Crescini, C., Idi, G., Artuso, A., Morganti, P., Repetti, F. (1991). 'Delivery after previous cesarean section. Experience with 173 patients'. *Minerva Ginecologica*, 43(11), pp. 513–18.

Conner, B.S. (1977). 'Teaching about Cesarean birth in traditional childbirth classes'. *Birth and the Family Journal*, 4, pp. 107–113.

Cotgrove, S.A., Norton, J.F. (1942). 'Cesarean section'. *Journal of the American Medical Association* (JAMA), 118(3), pp. 201–04.

Cox, B., Smith, E. (1982). 'The mother's self-esteem after a caesarean delivery'. *Maternal Child Nursing*, 7, pp. 309–14.

Cox, L.W. (1986). 'Breech presentation: a review of current practice'. *Midwifery*, 2(2), pp. 71–80.

Crafter, H. (1994). 'Forcible caesarean: a new direction in British maternity care? Thoughts on the case of Mrs S'. *Nursing Ethics*, 1(1), pp. 53–55.

Cranley, M.S., Hedahl, K.J., Pegg, S. (1983). 'Women's perceptions of vaginal and cesarean deliveries'. *Nursing Research*, 32, pp. 10–15.

Culp, R.E., Osofsky, H.J. (1989). 'Effects of cesarean delivery on parental depression, marital adjustment and mother-infant interaction'. *Birth*, 16(2), pp. 53–57.

Davis, K. (1994). 'Responsibilities of choice'. *Nursing Standard*, 8(44), p. 21.

Davis, L.G., Reidman, G.L., Sapiro, M., Minogue, J.P., Kazer, R.R. (1994). 'Cesarean section rates in low risk private patients managed by certified nurse-midwives and obstetricians'. *Journal of Nurse Midwifery*, 39(2), pp. 91–97.

Dean, S. (1986). 'Change the subject – I've had a caesarean'. *Nursing Times*, May 28, Midwives Journal, 66.

DeLee, J.B. (1913). *Principles and Practice of Obstetrics*. London: W.B. Saunders.

DeLee, J.B. (1942). 'Cesarean section'. *Journal of the American Medical Association*, 118(3), pp. 201–09.

DeMott, R.K., Sandmire, H.F. (1992). 'The Green Bay cesarean section study. II. The physician factor as a determinant of cesarean birth rates for failed labor'. *American Journal of Obstetrics and Gynecology*, 166(6 part 1), pp. 1799–1806.

Derom, R., Patel, N.B., Thiery, M. (1987). 'Implications of increasing rates of Caesarean section'. In: Studd, J. (Ed). *Progress in Obstetrics and Gynaecology*. Vol. VI, Edinburgh: Churchill Livingstone.

Department of Health and Social Security (1982). *Report on Confidential Enquiries into Maternal Deaths in the United Kingdom*. London: HMSO.

Department of Health (1991). *Report on Confidential Enquiries into Maternal Deaths in the United Kingdom*. London: HMSO.

Department of Health (1993). *Changing Childbirth: The Report of the Expert Maternity Group (Cumberledge Report)*. London: HMSO.

Department of Health (1994). *Report on Confidential Enquiries into Maternal Deaths in the United Kingdom 1988–1990*. London: HMSO.

Dillon, W.P., Choate, J.W., Nusbaum, M.L., McCarthy, M.A., McCall, M., Rosen, M. (1992). 'Obstetric care and cesarean birth rates: A program to monitor quality of care'. *Obstetrics and Gynecology*, 80(5), pp. 731–37.

Domnick Pierre, K., Vayda, E., Lomas, J., Endin, M.W., Hannah, W.J., Anderson, G.M. (1991). 'Obstetrical attitudes and practices before and after the Canadian Consensus Conference Statement on cesarean birth'. *Social Science and Medicine*, 32(11), pp. 1283–89.

Eakes, M. (1990) 'Economic considerations for epidural anesthesia in childbirth'. *Nursing Economics*, 8(5), pp. 329–32.

Egbert, L.D., Battit, G.E., Welch, C.E., Bartlett, M.K. (1964). 'Reduction of postoperative pain by encouragement and instruction of patients'. *New England Journal of Medicine*, 270, pp. 825–827.

Ehrenreich, B., English, D. (1979). *For Her Own Good, 150 Years of the Experts' Advice to Women*. London: Pluto.

Engelkes, E., van Roosmalen, J. (1992.) 'The value of symphyseotomy compared with caesarean section in cases of obstructed labour'. *Social Science and Medicine*, 35(6), pp. 789–93.

Enkin, M.W. (1977). 'Having a section is having a baby'. *Birth and the Family Journal*, 4, pp. 99–103.

Entwisle, D.R., Alexander, K.L. (1987). 'Long-term effects of cesarean delivery on parents' beliefs and children's schooling'. *Developmental Psychology*, 23, pp. 676–82.

Ever-Hadani, P., Seidman D.S., Manor, O., Harlap, S. (1994). 'Breast feeding in Israel: Maternal factors associated with choice and duration'. *Journal of Epidemiology and Community Health*, 48(3), pp. 281–85.

Evrad, J.R., Gold, E.M. (1977). 'Cesarean section and maternal mortality in Rhode Island – incidence and risk factors 1965–1975'. *Obstetrics and Gynecology*, 50, pp. 594–97.

Faundes, A., Cecatti, J.G. (1993). 'Which policy for caesarian section in Brazil? An analysis of the trends and consequences'. *Health Policy and Planning*, 8, pp. 33–42.

Fawcett, J. (1981). 'Needs of cesarean birth parents'. *Journal of Obstetric, Gynaecological and Neonatal Nursing*, 10, pp. 372–76.

Fawcett, J. (1990). 'Preparation for caesarean childbirth: Derivation of a nursing intervention from the Roy Adaptation Model'. *Journal of Advanced Nursing*, 15, pp. 1418–1425.

Fawcett, J., Burritt, J. (1985). 'An exploratory study of antenatal preparation for cesarean birth'. *Journal of Obstetric, Gynecological and Neonatal Nursing*, 14(3), pp. 224–30.

Fawcett, J., Henklein, J.C. (1987). 'Antenatal education for cesarean birth: extension of a field test'. *Journal of Obstetric, Gynaecologic and Neonatal Nursing*, 16(1), pp. 61–65.

Fawcett, J., Pollio, N., Tully, A. (1992). 'Women's perceptions of cesarean and vaginal delivery, another look'. *Research in Nursing and Health*, 15, pp. 439–46.

Fawcett, J., Pollio, N., Tully, A., Baron, M., Henklein, J.C., Jones, R.C. (1993). 'Effects of information on adaptation to cesarean birth'. *Nursing Research*, 42(1), pp. 49–53.

Finney, Rev. P.A. (1935). *Moral Problems in Hospital Practice*. Fifth Edition. London: B. Herder Book Company.

Flint, C. (1994). 'Hailing a new philosophy'. *Nursing Standard*, 8(20), p. 20.

Foote, A.J. (1995). 'External cephalic version from 34 weeds under tocolysis: factors influencing success'. *Journal of Obstetrics and Gynaecology*, 21(2), pp. 127–32.

Forman, M.R., Berendest, H.W., Lewando-Hundt, G., Sarov, B., Naggan, L. (1991). 'Perinatal factors influencing infant feeding practices at birth: the Bedouin Infant Feeding Study'. *Paediatric and Perinatal Epidemiology*, 5(2), pp. 168–80.

Francome, C. (1990). *Sane New World, Replacing Values*. Middlesex: Carla Publications.

Francome, C. (1994). *Caesarean Birth in Britain (1994 Supplement)*. Middlesex University.

Francome, C., Huntingford, P.J. (1980). 'Births by caesarean section in the United States of America and Britain'. *Journal of Biosocial Science*, 12, pp. 353–62.

Francome, C., Savage, W., Churchill, H., Lewison, H. (1993). *Caesarean Birth in Britain*. Cambridge: Middlesex University.

Frazer, M.I. (1987). 'So great a cruelty – historical aspects of caesarean section'. *Midwifery*, 3, pp. 72–74.

Freda, M.C. (1994). 'Commentary on six myths of maternal posture during labor'. *AWHONN's Women's Health Nursing Scan*, 8(2), p. 13.

Fullerton, J.T., Severino, R. (1992). 'In-hospital care for low-risk childbirth: comparison with results from the National Birth Center Study'. *Journal of Nurse Midwifery*, 37(5), pp. 331–40.

Garel, M., Lelong, N., Marchand, A., Kaminski, M. (1990). 'Psychosocial consequences of caesarean childbirth: A four-year follow-up study'. *Early Human Development*, 21(2), pp. 105–14.

Gatterer, G., Kubinger, K.D. (1985). 'Intellectual and physical damage following breech delivery'. *Zeitschrift fur Experimentelle und Angewandte Psychologie*, 32(3), pp. 384–99.

Goh, J.T., Johnson, C.M., Gregora, M.G. (1993). 'External cephalic version at term'. *Australian and New Zealand Journal of Obstetrics and Gynaecology*, 33(4), pp. 364–66.

Goldman, G., Pineault, R., Potvin, L., Blais, R., Bilodeau, H. (1993). 'Factors influencing the practice of vaginal birth after cesarean section'. *American Journal of Public Health*, 83(8), pp. 1104–08.

Goteborgs, U. (1987). 'Cesarean children in Sweden: Effects on the mother and father - infant relationship'. *Infant Mental Health Journal*, 8(2), pp. 91–99.

Gottlieb, S.E., Barrett, D.E. (1986). 'Effects of unanticipated cesarean section on mothers, infants and their interaction in the first month of life'. *Journal of Developmental and Behavioral Pediatrics*, 7, p. 180.

Graham, H., Oakley, A. (1981). 'Competing ideologies of reproduction: medical and maternal perspectives on pregnancy'. In: Roberts, H. (Ed). *Women, Health and Reproduction*. London: Routledge and Kegan Paul.

Greene, P.G., Zeichner, A., Roberts, N.L., Callahan, E.J., Granados, J.L. (1989). 'Preparation for caesarean delivery: a multicomponent analysis of treatment outcome'. *Journal of Consultants in Clinical Psychology*, 57, pp. 484–87.

Greenhill, J. (1931). *Surgery, Gynaecology and Obstetrics*. 53, p. 547.

Guillemin, J. (1981). 'Babies by cesarean: who chooses, who controls?'. *The Hastings Center Report*, 11, pp. 15–18.

Guillimeau, J. (1612). *Childbirth*. London: A. Hatfield.

Hare, S. (1838). 'Objections to the caesarean operation'. *The Lancet*, 2, pp. 702–03.

Hall, M.H., Campbell, D.M., Fraser, C., Lemon, J. (1989). 'Mode of delivery and future fertility'. *British Journal of Obstetrics and Gynaecology*, 96, pp. 1297–1303.

Hamilton, A. (1803). *Outlines of the Theory and Practice of Midwifery*. 5th Edition. Edinburgh: T. Kay.

Hannah, P., Adams, D., Lee, A., Glover, V. (1992). 'Links between early post-partum mood and postnatal depression'. *Journal of Psychiatry*, 160, pp. 777–80.

Hansell, R.S., McMurray, K.B., Huey, G.R. (1990). 'Vaginal birth after two or more cesarean sections: A five-year experience'. *Birth*, 17(3), pp. 146–50.

Hare, S. (1838). 'Objections to the caesarean operation'. *The Lancet*, 2, pp. 702–03.

Harris, R.P. (1888). *International Journal of Medical Science*, 95, p. 150.

Haultain, W.F.T. (1933). *Transcripts of the Obstetric Society of Edinburgh*. 54, p. 121.

Health Committee (1992). *Maternity Services, House of Commons, Second Report*. London: HMSO.

Hemminki, E. (1991). 'Long term maternal health effects after caesarean section'. *Journal of Epidemiology and Community Health*, 45, pp. 24–28.

Hemminki, E., Kojo-Austin, H., Malin, M., Koponwn, P. (1992). 'Variation in obstetric interventions by midwife'. *Scandinavian Journal of Caring Sciences*, 6(2), pp. 81–86.

Hillan, E. (1991). 'Caesarean section: psychological effects'. *Nursing Standard*, 5(50), pp. 30–33.

Hillan, E. (1992). 'Research and audit, Women's views of caesarean section'. In: Roberts, H. (Ed). *Women's Health Matters*. London: Routledge.

Holland, E. (1921a). 'Methods of performing caesarean section'. *The Journal of Obstetrics and Gynaecology of the British Empire*, Index to volume 28, pp. 349–57.

Holland, E. (1921b). 'The results of a collective investigation into caesarean sections performed in Great Britain and Ireland from the year 1911 to 1920 inclusive'. *The Journal of Obstetrics and Gynaecology of the British Empire*, Index to volume 28, pp. 358–82.

Holmes, R.W. (1915). *Surgery, Gynecology and Obstetrics*, 21, p. 636.

Holt, M. (1986). 'Ghosts from the past'. *Nursing Times*, August 13, p. 60.

How, K., Foley, M., Stronge, J. (1995). 'Nulliparous caesarean section in the home of active management of labour'. *Australian and New Zealand Journal of Obstetrics and Gynaecology*, 35(1), pp. 12–15.

Hughes, D., Parker, O. (1986). 'Paving the way to reform'. *Nursing Times*, May 28, Midwives Journal, p. 62.

Hull, J. (1798). *A Defence of the Caesarean Operation*. Manchester: R. & W. Dean.

Hull, J. (1799). *Observations on Mr. Simmons' Reflection on the Propriety of Performing the Caesarean Operation, with a Defense of the Caesarean Operation*. Manchester.

Huntingford, P. (1985). *Birth Right, The Parents' Choice*. London: BBC.

Hurst, M., Summey, P. (1984). 'Childbirth and social class: The case of caesarean delivery'. *Social Science and Medicine*, 18(8), pp. 621–31.

Inch, S. (1985). *Birthrights, A Parents' Guide to Modern Childbirth*. London: Hutchinson.

Inch, S. (1986). 'When the midwife misses out'. *Nursing Times*, May 28, Midwives Journal, p. 67.

Iglesias, S., Burn, R., Saunders, L.D. (1991). 'Reducing the cesarean section rate in a rural community hospital'. *Canadian Medical Association Journal*, 145(11), pp. 1459–64.

Inlander, C.B. (1990). 'Truth in medicine'. *Nursing Economics*, 8(3), pp. 196,198.

Janke, J.R. (1988). 'Breastfeeding duration following cesarean and vaginal births'. *Journal of Nurse Midwifery*, Jul–Aug, 33(4), pp. 159–64.

Janowitz, B., Wallace, S., Araujo, L. (1984). 'Method of payment and the cesarean birth rate in a hospital in North-east Brazil'. *Journal of Health Politics, Policy and Law*, 9, pp. 515–526.

Journal of the American Medical Association (1794). 115, 1942.

Kanto, J., Laine, M., Vuorisalo, A., Salonen, M. (1990). 'Pre-operative preparation'. *Nursing Times*, 86(20), pp. 39–41.

Kearney, M.H., Cronenwett, L.R., Reinhardt, R. (1990). 'Cesarean delivery and breastfeeding outcomes'. *Birth*, 17(2), pp. 97–103.

Keeler, E.B., Brodie, M. (1993). 'Economic incentives in the choice between vaginal delivery and cesarean section'. *Milbank Quarterly*, 71(3), pp. 365–404.

Kennel, J.H., Jerauld, R., Wolfe, H., Chesler, D., Kreger, N.C., McAlpine, W., Steffa, M., Klaus, M.H. (1974). 'Maternal behaviour one year after early and extended post-partum contact'. *Developmental Medicine and Child Neurology*, 16, pp. 172–79.

Kerr, J.M.M. (1921). 'Indication for caesarean section'. *The Journal of Obstetrics and Gynaecology of the British Empire*, Index to volume 28, pp. 338–49.

Kerr, J.M.M. (1937). *Operative Obstetrics*. 4th Edition. London: Bailliere Tindall and Cox Ltd.

Kirkham, M. (1986). 'A feminist perspective on midwifery'. In: Webb, C. (Ed). *Feminist Practice in Women's Health Care*. Chichester: John Wiley and Sons.

Kitzenger, S. (1980). *Pregnancy and Childbirth*. London: Penguin.

Klaus, M.H., Kennell, J.H. (1982). *Parent–Infant Bonding*. London: The CV Mosby Company.

Krishnamurthy, S., Fairlie, F., Cameron, A.D., Walker, J.J., Mackenzie, J.R. (1991). 'The role of postnatal X-ray pelvimetry after caesarean section in the management of subsequent delivery'. *British Journal of Obstetrics and Gynaecology*, 98, pp. 716–18.

Lagercrantz, H., Slotkin, T.A. (1986). 'The "stress" of being born'. *Scientific American*, 254(4), pp. 100–07.

Lancet (1851a). 'Proceedings of the meeting of the royal medical and chirurgical society'. January 28, 1851, 1, pp. 152–55.

Lancet (1851b). 'Proceedings of the meeting of the royal medical and chirurgical society'. February 11, 1851, 1, pp. 204–10.

Lancet (1891). 'Modern methods of caesarean section'. April.

Laufer, A., Hodenius, V., Friedman, et al. (1987). 'Vaginal birth after saesarean section: Nurse - midwifery management'. *Journal of Nurse-Midwifery*, 32,1, pp. 41–47.

Lelong, N., Kaminski, M. (1987) .'Psychological consequences of caesarean childbirth in primiparas'. *Journal of Psychosomatic Obstetrics and Gynaecology*, 6, pp. 197–209.

LoCicero, A. K. (1993). 'Explaining excessive rates of cesareans and other childbirth interventions: contributions from contemporary theories of gender and psychosocial development'. *Social Science and Medicine*, 37(10), pp. 1261–269.

Lomas, J., Enkin, M. (1989). 'Variations in operative delivery rates'. In: Chalmers, I., Enkin, M., Keirse, M. (Eds). *Effective Care in Pregnancy and Childbirth*. Oxford: Oxford University Press.

Lull, C.B. (1933). *American Journal of Obstetrics and Gynecology*. 25, 426.

Lydon-Rochelle, M. (1995). 'Cesarean delivery rates in women cared for by certified nurse-midwives in the United States: a review'. *Birth Issues in Perinatal Care and Education*, 22(4), pp. 211–19.

Lynch, M.A., Roberts, J. (1977). 'Predicting child abuse: signs of bonding failure in the maternity hospital'. *British Medical Journal*, 1, p. 624.

Macara, L.M., Murphy, K.W. (1994). 'The contribution of dystocia to the cesarean section rate'. *American Journal of Obstetrics and Gynecology*, 171(1), pp. 71–77.

MacArthur, C., Lewis, M., Knox, E.G. (1991). *Health after Childbirth*. London: HMSO.

Macdonald, R. (1990). 'Analgesia following caesarean section'. 103, pp. 202–04.

Macfarlane, A. (1984). 'Day of birth'. *The Lancet*, 2, p. 695.

Macfarlane, A., Mugford, M. (1986). 'An epidemic of caesareans?'. *Maternal and Child Health*, 11, pp. 38–42.

Macfarlane, A., Chamberlain, G. (1993). 'What is happening to caesarean section rates?'. *The Lancet*, 342, pp. 1005–06.

Macnair, P. (1992). 'Cutting both ways, the reasons behind the rising number of births by Caesarean section'. *The Guardian*, February, p. 18.

Maher, C.F., Cave, D.G., Haran, M.V. (1994). 'Caesarean section rate reduced'. *Australian and New Zealand Journal of Obstetrics and Gynaecology*, 34(4), pp. 389–92.

Marieskind, H.I. (1989). 'Cesarean section in the United States: has it changed since 1979?'. *Birth*, 16(4), pp. 196–202.

Martin, C. (1990). 'How do you count maternal satisfaction? A user-commissioned survey of maternity services'. In: Roberts, H. (Ed). *Women's Health Counts*. London: Routledge.

Marut, J.S., Mercer, R.T. (1979). 'Comparison of primiparas' perceptions of vaginal and cesarean births'. *Nursing Research*, 28, pp. 260–66.

Mathur, G.P., Pandey, P.K., Mathur, S., Sharma, S. (1993). 'Breastfeeding in babies delivered by cesarean section'. *Indian Pediatrics*, 30(11), pp. 1285–90.

May, K.A., Sollidd, D.T. (1984). 'Unanticipated cesarean birth from the father's perspective'. *Birth*, 11, pp. 87–95.

McCusker, J., Harris, D.K., Hosmer, D.W. (1988). 'Association of electronic fetal monitoring during labour with cesarean section rate and with neonatal morbidity and mortality'. *American Journal of Public Health*, 78, pp. 1170–04.

McGarry, J.A. (1969). 'The management of patients previously delivered by caesarean section'. *Journal of Obstetrics and Gynaecology of the British Commonwealth*, 76, pp. 137–43.

McIlroy, L. (1932a). *Proceedings of the Royal Society of Medicine*. 26, p. 85.

McIlroy, L. (1932b). *British Medical Journal*. 10, p. 796.

McIlwaine, G.M., Cole, S.K., Macnaughton, M.C. (1985). 'The rising caesarean rate – A matter of concern?'. *Health Bulletin*, 43(6), pp. 301–05.

Menghetti, E., Marulli, P., Mucedola, G., Montaleone, M. (1994). 'The nutrition of the nursing mother in light of a study of 200 new mothers'. *Minerva Pediatrica*, 46(7–8), pp. 331–34.

Metcalfe, J. (1986). 'An image restored'. *Nursing Times*, May 28, Midwives Journal, p. 66.

Minkoff, H.L., Schwarcz, R.H. (1980). 'The rising cesarean rate – can it safely be reversed?'. *Obstetrics and Gynecology*, 56, pp. 135–43.

Moldin, P., Hökegárd, K-H., Nielsen, T.F. (1984). 'Caesarean section and maternal mortality in Sweden 1973–1979'. *Acta Obstetrics and Gynecology Scandanavia*, 63, pp. 7–11.

Molloy, B.G., Sheil, O., Duignan, N.M. (1987). 'Delivery after caesarean section: review of 2176 consecutive cases'. *British Medical Journal*, 294, pp. 1645–47.

Morgan, B.M., Aulakh, J.M., Barker, J.P., Reginald, P.W., Goroszeniuk, T., Trojanowski, A. (1984). 'Anaesthetic morbidity following caesarean section under epidural or general anaesthesia'. *The Lancet*, 1, pp. 328–30.

Morgan, D. (1992). 'Whatever happened to consent?'. *New Law Journal*, 142, p. 1448.

Morton, S.C., Williams, M.S., Keeler, E.B., Gambone, J.C., Kahn, K.L. (1994). 'Effect of epidural analgesia for labor on the cesarean delivery rate'. *Obstetrics and Gynecology*, 83(6), pp. 1045–52.

Mukherjee, J., Bhattacharya, P.K., Lahiri, T.K., Samaddar, J.C., Mehta, R. (1993). 'Perinatal mortality in cesarean section: a disturbing picture of unfulfilled expectations'. *Journal of the Indian Medical Association*, 91(8), pp. 202–3.

Murray-Arthur, F., Correy, J.F. (1984). 'A review of primary caesarean sections in Tasmania'. *Australian and New Zealand Journal of Obstetrics and Gynaecology*, 24, pp. 242–5.

Myers, S.A., Gleicher, N. (1990). '1988 US cesarean-section rate: Good news or bad?'. *The New England Journal of Medicine*, 323(3), p. 200.

Nair, C. (1991). 'Trends in cesarean section deliveries in Canada'. *Health Reports*, 3(3), pp. 203–19.

National Institutes of Health (1981). *Cesarean Birth: Report of a Consensus Development Conference*. Bethesda, Maryland: NIH Publication No. 82–2067.

Nielsen, T.F., Hökegárd, K-H. (1984). 'Cesarean section and intraoperative surgical complications'. *Acta Obstetrics and Gynecology Scandanavia*, 63, pp. 103–8.

Nielsen, T.F., Ljungblad, U., Hagberg, H. (1989). 'Rupture and dehiscence of cesarean section scar during pregnancy and delivery'. *American Journal of Obstetrics and Gynecology*, 160, pp. 569–73.

Newell, F.S. (1921). *Cesarean Section*. New York, London: D. Appleton and Co.

Nolan, M. (1990). 'Normal delivery after caesarean section'. *Nursing Times*, Aug. 8, Vol. 86, 32, pp. 34–36.

Norman, P., Kostovcik, S., Lanning, A. (1993). 'Elective repeat cesarean sections: how many could be vaginal births?'. *Canadian Medical Association Journal*, 149(4), pp. 431–5.

Nöth, A. (1931). *Die Hebammenordnungen des XVIII. Jahrhunderts*. Medical Dissertations: Würzburg. (Midwife Ordinance of the Burggrafschaft Nürnberg).

Notzon, F.C., Placek, P.J., Taffel, S.M. (1987). 'Comparisons of national cesarean-section rates'. *The New England Journal of Medicine*, 316(7), pp. 386–9.

Notzon, F.C., Cnattingius, S., Bergsjo, P., Cole, S., Taffel, S., Irgens, L., Daltveit, A.K. (1994). 'Cesarean section delivery in the 1980s: international comparison by indication'. *American Journal of Obstetrics and Gynecology*, 170(2), pp. 495–504.

Oakley, A. (1980). *Women Confined*. Oxford: Martin Robertson & Co. Ltd.

Oakley, A., Richards, M. (1990). 'Women's experiences of caesarean delivery'. In: Garcia, J., Kilpatrick, R., Richards, M. (Eds). *The Politics of Maternity Care*. Oxford: Clarendon Press.

O'Brien, M. (1978). 'Home and hospital: a comparison of the experience of mothers having home and hospital confinements'. *Journal of the Royal College of General Practitioners*, 28, pp. 460–6.

O'Driscoll, K., Foley, M. (1983). 'Correlation of decrease in perinatal mortality and increase in Caesarean section rate'. *Obstetrics and Gynaecology*, 61(1), pp. 1–5.

O'Driscoll, K., Foley, M., MacDonald, D. (1984). 'Active management of labour as an alternative to cesarean section for dystocia'. *Obstetrics and Gynecology*, 63(4), pp. 485–90.

Olofsson, P., Rydhström, H. (1985). 'Twin delivery: How should the second twin be delivered?'. *American Journal of Obstetrics and Gynecology*, 153(5), pp. 479–81.

Onsrud, L., Onsrud, M. (1996). 'Increasing use of caesarean section, even in developing countries'. *Tidsskrift for Den Norske Laegeforening*, 116(1), pp. 67–71.

Padawer, J.A., Fagan, C., Janoff-Bulman, R., Strickland, B.R. (1988). 'Women's psychological adjustment following emergency cesarean versus vaginal delivery'. *Psychology of Women Quarterly*, 12, pp. 25–34.

Parer, J.T., Livingston, E.G. (1990). 'What is fetal distress?'. *American Journal of Obstetrics and Gynecology*, 162, pp. 1421–7.

Paterson, C.M., Saunders, N.J. St. G. (1991). 'Mode of delivery after one caesarean section: audit of current practice in a health region'. *British Medical Journal*, 303, pp. 818–20

Paul, R.H., Phelan, J.P., Yeh, S. (1985). 'Trial of labor in the patient with prior cesarean birth'. *American Journal of Obstetrics and Gynecology*, 151, pp. 297–304.

Peipert, J.F., Bracken M.B. (1993). 'Maternal age: an independent risk factor for cesarean delivery'. *Obstetrics and Gynecology*, 81(2), pp. 200–5.

Penso, C. (1994). 'Vaginal birth after cesarean section: an update on physician trends and patient perceptions [Review]'. *Current Opinion in Obstetrics and Gynecology*, 6(5), pp. 417–25.

Perez, P.G. (1989). 'The patient observer: What really led to these cesarean births?'. *Birth*, 16(3), pp. 130–9.

Phillips, A. (1983). *Your Body, Your Baby, Your Life*. London: Pandora Press.

Phillips, A., Rakusen, J. (1978). *Our Bodies Ourselves*. Harmondsworth: Penguin.

Phillips, R.N., Thornton, J., Gleicher, N. (1982). 'Physician bias in cesarean sections'. *Journal of the American Medical Association*, 248(9), pp. 1082–4.

Placek, P.J., Taffel, S.M., Moien, M. (1987). 'Cesarean rate increases in 1985'. *American Journal of Public Health*, 77, pp. 241–42.

Placek, P.J., Taffel, S.M. (1988). 'Vaginal Birth After Cesarean (VBAC) in the 1980s'. *American Journal of Public Health*, 78, pp. 512–15.

Plass, E.D. (1931). *American Journal of Obstetrics and Gynecology*, 22, 176.

Playfair, W.S. (1886). *The Science and Practice of Midwifery*. Smith, Elder and Company.

Porreco, R.P. (1985). 'High cesarean section rate: A new perspective'. *Obstetrics and Gynecology*, 65, pp. 307–11.

Radford, T. (1865). *Observations on the Caesarean Section and on Other Obstetric Operations*. London: T. Richards.

Ranjan, V. (1993). 'Obstetrics and the fear of litigation'. *Professional Care of Mother and Child*, 3(1), pp. 10–12.

Reichert, J.A., Baron, M., Fawcett, J. (1993). 'Changes in attitudes towards cesarean birth'. *Journal of Obstetric, Gynecologic and Neonatal Nursing*, 22(2), pp. 159–67.

Renwick, M.Y. (1991). *The Australian and New Zealand Journal of Obstetrics and Gynaecology*, 31(4), pp. 299–304.

Richards, M. (1979). 'Perinatal morbidity and mortality in private obstetric practice'. *The Journal of Maternal and Child Health*, 4(9), pp. 341–5.

Richards, M.P.M. (1983). 'Caesarean birth and the development of children'. *Midwife, Health Visitor and Community Nurse*, 19(9), pp. 368–72.

Rockenschaub, A. (1990) 'Technology-free obstetrics at the Semmelweis Clinic'. *The Lancet*, 335, p. 977.

Rodin, T.G., Harman, J.S., Hanson, D.A. (1993). 'Nurses' care during labour: its effect on the cesarean birth rate of healthy, nulliparous women'. *Birth*, 20(1), pp. 14–21.

Romalis, S. (1985). 'Struggle between providers and recipients: the case of birth practices'. In: Lewin, E., Olesen, V. (Eds). *Women, Health and Healing, Toward A New Perspective*. London: Tavistock.

Rooks, J.P., Weatherby, N.L., Ernst, E.K.M., Stapleton, S., Rosen, D., Rosenfield, A. (1989). 'Outcomes of care in birth centres'. *New England Journal of Medicine*, 321; pp. 1804–11.

Routh, A. (1911). *Journal of Obstetrics and Gynaecology of the British Empire*, 19, pp. 1–25.

Royal College of Midwives (1991). *Successful Breastfeeding*. (Second edition). London: Livingstone.

Rydhström, H., Ingemarsson, I., Ohrlander, S. (1990). 'Lack of correlation between a high caesarean section rate and improved prognosis for low–birthweight twins (<2500g)'. *British Journal of Obstetrics and Gynaecology*, 97, pp. 229–33.

Sakala, C. (1993). 'Midwifery care and out-of-hospital birth settings: How do they reduce unnecessary cesarean section births?'. *Social Science and Medicine*, 37(10), pp. 1233–1250.

Sanchez-Ramos, L., Kaunitz, A.M., Peterson, H.B., Martinez-Schnell, B., Thompson, R.J. (1990). 'Reducing cesarean sections at a teaching hospital'. *American Journal of Obstetrics and Gynecology*, 163, pp. 1081–8.

Sande, H.A. (1993). 'External cephalic version of breech presentation'. *Tidsskrift for Den Norske Laegeforening*, 113(25), pp. 3153–4.

Santamera, S.A., Gutierrez S.J.M. (1994). 'Evolution of cesarean section rates in Spain: 1984–1988'. *Gaceta Sanitaria*, 8(44), pp. 209–14.

Sargent, C., Stark, N. (1987). 'Surgical birth: Interpretations of cesarean delivery among private hospital patients and nursing staff'. *Social Science and Medicine*, 25(12), pp. 1269–76.

Sargent, C., Stark, N (1989). 'Childbirth education and childbirth models: Parental perspectives on control, anaesthesia, and technological intervention in the birth process'. *Medical Anthropology Quarterly*, 3, pp. 36–51.

Savage, W. (1986). 'Changing attitudes to intervention'. *Nursing Times*, May 28, Midwives Journal, p. 63.

Savage, W., Francome, C. (1993). 'British caesarean section rates: have we reached a plateau?'. *British Journal of Obstetrics and Gynaecology*, 100(5), pp. 403–6.

Savage, W. (1994). 'Commentary'. In: Francome, C. (Ed). *Caesarean Birth in Britain* (1994 Supplement). Middlesex University.

Schroeder, C. (1873). *Manual of Midwifery*. Third Edition, translated by C.H. Carter, London: Churchill.

Seguin, L., Therrien, R., Champagne, F., Larouche, D. (1989). 'The components of women's satisfaction with maternity care'. *Birth*, 16(3), pp. 109–13.

Sepkowitz, S. (1992). 'Birth weight–specific fetal deaths and neonatal mortality and the rising cesarean section rate'. *Journal of the Oklahoma State Medical Association*, 85(5), pp. 236–41.

Shakespeare, W. (1605). *Macbeth*.

Shapiro, M.C., Najman, J.M., Chang, A., Keeping, J.D., Morrison, J., Western J.S. (1983). 'Information control and the exercise of power in the obstetrical encounter'. *Social Science and Medicine*, 17(3), pp. 139–46.

Shearer, E.L. (1989). 'Commentary: Does cesarean delivery affect the parents?'. *Birth*, 16, pp. 57–8.

Shearer, E.L. (1993). 'Cesarean section: medical benefits and costs [review]'. *Social Science and Medicine*, 37(10), pp. 1223–31.

Shepperd McClain, C. (1990). 'The making of a medical tradition: Vaginal birth after cesarean'. *Social Science and Medicine*, 31(2), pp. 203–10.

Shorter, E. (1982). *A History of Women's Bodies*. London: Allen Lane.

Shulte, A.J. (1917). quoted in *The Critic and Guide*. New York, p. 52.

Simmons, W. (1798). 'Reflection on the propriety of performing the caesarean operation'. *The Medical and Physical Journal*, 2, p. 231.

Simons, C.J.R., Ritchie, S.K., Mullet, M.D. (1992). 'Relationships between parental ratings of infant temperament, risk status and delivery method'. *Journal of Pediatric Health Care*, 6(5 part 1), pp. 240–5.

Smellie, W. (1766). *A Treatise on the Theory and Practice of Midwifery*. 5th edition. London: D Wilton.

Smith, A.M. (1990). 'Obstetrics and technology'. *The Lancet* (letter), 336, pp. 510–11.

Stafford, R.S. (1990). 'Cesarean section use and source of payment: an analysis of California hospital discharge abstracts'. *American Journal of Public Health*, 80(3), pp. 313–5.

Stafford, R.S. (1991). 'The impact of nonclinical factors on repeat cesarean section'. *Journal of the American Medical Association*, 265(1), pp. 59–63.

Stafford, R.S., Sullivan, S.D., Gardner, L.B. (1993). 'Trends in cesarean section use in California, 1983 to 1990'. *American Journal of Obstetrics and Gynecology.*, 168(4), pp. 1297–302.

Stewart, D. (1747). 'The caesarean operation done with success by a midwife'. *Medical Essays and Observations*, 3(1), pp. 360–2.

Stewart, D. (1771). *Edinburgh Medical Essays and Observations*, 5, p. 37.

Taffel, S.M., Placek, P.J., Moien, M. (1985). 'One-fifth of 1983 United States' births by cesarean section'. *American Journal of Public Health*, 75, p. 190.

Taffel, S.M., Placek, P.J., Moien, M. (1990). '1988 US cesarean-section rate at 24.7 per 100 births - A plateau?'. *The New England Journal of Medicine*, 323(3), pp. 199–200.

Taffel, S.M., Placek, P.J., Moinen, M., Kosary, C.L. (1991). '1989 U.S. cesarean section rate steadies – VBAC rate rises to nearly one in five'. *Birth*, 18 (2), pp. 73–7.

Taffel, S.M., Placek, P.J., Kosary, C.L. (1992). 'US cesarean section rates 1990: An update'. *Birth*, 19(1), pp. 21–2.

Taffel, S.M. (1994). 'Cesarean delivery in the United States, 1990'. *Vital and Health Statistics. Series 21, Data on Natality, Marriage and Divorce*, (51), pp. 1–24.

Tariq, T.A., Korejo, R. (1993). 'Evaluation of the role of craniotomy in developing countries'. *Journal of the Pakistan Medical Association*, 43(2), pp. 30–2.

Tay, S.K., Tsakok, F.H., Ng, C.S. (1992). 'The use of intradepartmental audit to contain cesarean section rate'. *International Journal of Gynaecology and Obstetrics*, 39(2), pp. 99–103.

Tenon, J.R. (1788). *Memoirs of the Hospital of Paris*. Paris.

Thoms, H. (1935). *Classical Contributions to Obstetrics and Gynaecology*. Springfield, Illinois: Charles C. Thomas.

Thorpe-Beeston, J.G., Banfield, P.J., Saunders, N.J. St.G. (1992). 'Outcome of breech delivery at term'. *British Medical Journal*, 305, pp. 746–7.

Thorp, J.A., McNitt, J.D., Leppert, P.C. (1990). 'Effects of epidural analgesia: some questions and answers'. *Birth*, 17(3), pp. 157–62.

Treffers, P.E., Pel, M. (1993). 'The rising trend for caesarean birth, Britain could learn from the Netherlands'. *British Medical Journal*, 307, pp. 1017–18.

Trowell, J. (1983). 'Emergency caesarean section: a research study of the mother/child relationship of a group of women admitted expecting a normal vaginal delivery'. *Child Abuse and Neglect*, 7, p. 387.

Trowell, J. (1986). 'Emotional effects of a caesarean'. *Nursing Times*, May 28, Midwives Journal, p. 64.

Trowell, J. (1989). 'Psychological effects of lower section caesarean'. *Midwife, Health Visitor and Community Nurse*, 25, pp. 22–24.

Tulman, L.J. (1986). 'Initial handling of newborn infants by vaginally and cesarean-delivered mothers'. *Nursing Research*, 35(5), pp. 296–300.

Tulman, L., Fawcett, J. (1991). 'Recovery from childbirth: looking back six months after delivery'. *Health Care for Women International*, 12(3), pp. 341–50.

Tussing, A.D., Wojtowycz, M.A. (1993). 'The effect of physician characteristics on clinical behaviour: cesarean section in New York State'. *Social Science and Medicine*, 37(10), pp. 1251–1260.

Tyler Smith, W. (1856). 'A course of lectures on the theory and practice of obstetrics'. *The Lancet*, 2, pp. 639–41.

Urquhart, D.R., Grieve, R.M.K., Geals, M.F. (1987). 'The rising caesarean section rate – a year's audit to assess the trend'. *Health Bulletin*, 45, pp. 316–28.

Van Roosmalen, J., van der Does, C.D. (1995). 'Caesarean birth rates worldwide. A search for determinants'. *Tropical and Geographical Medicine*, 47(1), pp. 19–22.

Vanderfuhr, F. (1826). 'Caesarean section successfully performed, both mother and child having been saved'. *The Lancet*, 9, p. 388.

Walmsley, K., Hobbs, L. (1994). 'Vaginal birth after lower segment caesarean section'. *Modern Midwife*, 4(4), pp. 20–1.

Wakley, T. (1838). *The Lancet* (editorial), 2, p. 703.

Webster, L.A., Daling, J.R., McFarlane, C., Ashley, D., Warren, C.W. (1992). 'Prevalence and determinants of caesarean section in Jamaica'. *Journal of Biosocial Science*, 24(4), pp. 515–25.

White, E., Shy, K.K., Daling, J.R. (1985). 'An investigation of the relationship between cesarean section birth and respiratory distress syndrome of the newborn'. *American Journal of Epidemiology*, 121, pp. 651–53.

Wilson, J.F. (1981). 'Behavioral preparation for surgery. Benefit or harm?'. *Journal of Behavioral Medicine*, 4, pp. 79–102.

Woodcraft, E. (1988). 'Bringing the arm of the law into the delivery-room. The right not to have a caesarean'. *The Listener*, February, pp. 14–15.

World Health Organization (1985). 'Appropriate technology for birth'. *The Lancet*, 2, pp. 436–7.

Young, J.H. (1944). *Caesarean Section: The history and development of the operation from the earliest times*. London: H.K. Lewis and Co. Ltd.

Zahniser, S.C., Kendrick, J.S., Franks, A.L., Saftlas, A.F. (1992). 'Trends in obstetric operative procedures 1980 to 1987'. *American Journal of Public Health*, 82(10), pp. 1340–4.

Zhang, J., Bowes, W.A., Fortney, J.A. (1993). 'Efficacy of external cephalic version: a review'. *Obstetrics and Gynecology*, 82(2), pp. 306–12.

Ziadeh, S.M., Sunna, E.I. (1995). 'Decreased cesarean birth rates and improved perinatal outcome: a seven–year study'. *Birth: Issues in Perinatal Care and Education*, 22(3), pp. 144–7.

Appendix I

Dr. Helen Churchill
the Manchester Metropolitan University
Hassall Road, Alsager,
Stoke-on-Trent, ST7 2HL

0161 247 5422

CAESAREAN SECTION QUESTIONNAIRE

I am interested in finding out how women feel about having a baby by caesarean. This study is being conducted as part of a major project on caesarean birth. The results of the study will be included in a new book entitled *Caesarean Section: Experience, Practice and History* to be published next year.

I am a Senior Lecturer and researcher at the Manchester Metropolitan University and as such am independent of this hospital. The questionnaires are anonymous. You do not have to fill in this questionnaire if you decide not to. If you would like to participate in the study please complete the attached questionnaire and return it to one of the nursing staff.

Thank you for your time and co-operation.

Yours sincerely,

Dr. Helen Churchill, B.A. (Hons.), Ph.D.
Co-author of *Caesarean Birth in Britain* (1993).

Instructions
Please tick the appropriate boxes for your answers.
If you have given birth by caesarean more than once, please answer the questions in relation to your most recent operation.

Please use the reverse of this letter for any additional comments you may have on giving birth by caesarean. If there is insufficient space please attach a separate sheet or write to me at the university.

Appendix II

CAESREAN SECTION QUESTIONNAIRE

About the operation

1. Was this caesarean section planned before hand (elective) ☐

   or done as an emergency? ☐

2. What reason(s) were you given for performing the caesarean operation? You may have been given more than one explanation so please tick the answers that apply to you.

☐ Baby too big for my pelvis	☐ Baby was distressed (fetal distress)
☐ Bleeding before birth	☐ Labour taking a long time (cervix not dilating)
☐ Baby in breech position	☐ Baby lying across my womb (transverse lie)
☐ Cord prolapse	☐ Cord around baby's neck
☐ Baby was small for dates	☐ I had diabetes
☐ I had a previous caesarean	☐ My blood pressure was high
☐ Because of my age	☐ Other reason (please specify).... ....

3. How many weeks pregnant were you when your baby was born?...........

4. What type of anaesthetic were you given?

   Epidural ☐ Spinal ☐ General ☐

5. Did you have a partner/birth companion present for the delivery?

   Yes ☐ No ☐

About your feelings and experience

6. Did you ask to have a caesarean section?   Yes ☐   No ☐

   If yes, why?...

7. At the time did you understand why a caesarean section was needed?

   Yes ☐   No ☐   Can't remember ☐

8. Before the were able to find out all you wanted to know about *your* condition?

   Yes ☐   No ☐

9. Were you kept informed of the treatment you were being given?

   Yes ☐   No ☐

   If no, what would you like to have been told?................................

   ....

10. Before the operation were you able to find out all you wanted to know about your *baby's* condition?

    Yes ☐   No ☐

11. Do you feel that you were kept fully informed about your baby's condition?

    Yes ☐   No ☐

    If no, what would like to have been told?....................................

    ....

12. Do you consider that you suffered as a result of having a caesarean?

    Yes ☐   No ☐

    If yes, why?...

13. After the caesarean did you feel pain in the wound more or less than expected?

    More than expected ☐   As expected ☐   Less than expected ☐

14. What else did you feel after the operation?

    Happy ☐   Tired ☐   Weak ☐   Relieved ☐   Sick ☐   Well ☐

    Depressed ☐   Other ☐ (please specify)....................................

    ....

About your baby

15. How much did your baby weigh at birth?......................................

16. Did you see your baby as soon as she/he was born?

    Yes ☐   No ☐   Can't remember ☐

17. Was your baby taken to intensive care/Special Care Baby Unit?

    Yes ☐   No ☐

    If yes, for how long?...

18. Did your baby need to be in an incubator?

    Yes ☐   No ☐

    If yes, for how long?...

About your relationship with your baby

19. Do you feel that the caesarean has had an effect on your ability to bond with your baby?

    Yes ☐   No ☐

    If yes, in what way(s)?...

20. Did you want to breastfeed your baby?   Yes ☐ No ☐ Unsure ☐

    If *no*, was this because:

    ☐ you are not keen on breastfeeding   ☐ you had no milk

    ☐ you changed your mind   ☐ you have inverted nipples

    ☐ you couldn't express the milk   ☐ you felt too ill

    ☐ your baby was ill   ☐ baby wouldn't take to breastfeeding

    ☐ you want to share the feeding   ☐ you think breastfeeding is inconvenient

    ☐ you prefer bottle feeding   ☐ previous failure with breastfeeding

    ☐ other (please specify)..

    ....

21. Do you feel that the caesarean has had an effect on your ability to breastfeed your baby?

Yes ☐   No ☐

If yes, in what way(s)?...

....

Now some questions about you

Age......... Number of times you have given birth (including this time).........

Your job or previous job..

Your partner's job (if applicable)..

Index